Sacred Awakening

Healing on my journey of cancer
through faith, family and gratitude

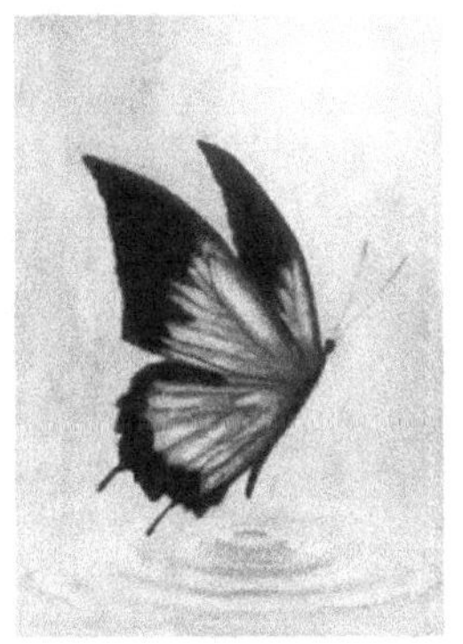

Amber Rae Strong

Sacred Awakening
Healing on my journey of cancer through faith, family and gratitude

---

To reach out to Amber:

www.amberraestrong.com

Follow on Instagram: @amber.rae.strong

Connect on Facebook: www.facebook.com/amberraestrong

Author Blog Site: https://fightlikeagirl333.wordpress.com

ISBN: 9781797733739 Paperback Third Edition
First Edition published June 2018

Front cover photo credit; Kim Acer Photography
Butterfly art courtesy; Emmylou Aurora Shine
Select photos within text courtesy; Kim Acer

In honor of Saint Rita of Cascia,
Patroness of the Impossible
For hearing my prayers, for guiding me through the
process of writing this book, for being an ever vigilant
guardian angel on my shoulder.
Grazie Mille

For Dominic and Izabella
You were the strength that pulled me through so
many days.
I love you more than you will ever know.

For those who have lost their lives to cancer;
Grandpa Teddy, Aunt Anne (Mia), Aunt Linda and
Marge.

For Millie; cancer took you away much too soon
beautiful. It could never dim the light of your
memory. You are loved and missed by many.

For the brave warriors who fought their way through
to survivorship; Uncle D, Courtney, Krissy M. and
the late Helen Barbacki.

For the cancer patients of the world, those newly
diagnosed, currently going through treatment or
losing hope - there is unimaginable strength within
you, have faith. You are never alone.

ACKNOWLEDGEMENTS

To my mother, Theresa.
For every trip to chemo, we made together, in the snow and
freezing New England weather. For every hug, for every day you
took off from work to look after Dom and Izzy, when I was too
sick to look after myself. For your guidance, strength and selfless
sacrifice - I cannot thank you enough and I love you so much
for the woman you have been, continue to be and for all you are
to me and your grandchildren. I'm so thankful to call you Mom.

To my father, Randy.
For every spaghetti dinner you cooked, for every baseball game
and practice you brought Dominic to. For every time you said
you were "in the area" and really weren't but stopped by anyway
because you were so worried about me, knowing I was too
proud to ask for help. For every night you got the kids to bed
for me or bought groceries to fill our bellies - you are my
HERO and I love you always.

To Dominic and Izabella, my "sun and stars"
and the "moon of my life."
Without both of you, there would be no me here today to share
my story. You were constant sources of strength when I was at
my weakest. The unconditional love you provided daily was
medicine for my soul.

Thank you Dom for making me laugh until my belly hurt. For
being such an amazing older brother to your sister, even if she
does drive you mental half the time. For random hugs and even
for days that weren't always easy because those too drove me to
find the strength to carry on. There is greatness within you,
always remember that.

Thank you Izzy for lighting up my life with your laughter. For every time you looked at me and said "Huggy, Mommy?"
For girl's day makeovers, movie night snuggles and the sassy comments you make that bring me to tears of laughter.
You are fierce little one, never ever change that.

To my siblings; Kim, Krissy, Matt, Nate and Aaron - I adore each of you. Thank you for supporting me emotionally, for providing laughter, love, sister sleepovers and countless family gatherings.

Thank you, Nate and Aaron, for venturing all the way from Florida to sit with me through hours of chemo and for being such good sports when I captured photos of you asleep in the chair.

Thank you, Kimmy, for looking after Dom and Izzy when I was in the hospital. Thank you for ensuring my taste buds weren't tormented by flavorless hospital food, time and time again.
Thank you for hosting a magical night out after treatment was complete, that allowed me to celebrate life with some most extraordinary women. For being an extraordinary woman yourself, whom I look up to and admire tremendously Love you to the moon and back sister.

Thank you, Emmylou, for your gift of designing the back cover art. For helping me step into my own greatness by "looking at things logically," helping me heal past pain and being my soul sister.
You may not have been part of my chemo journey then, but you are most certainly part of my journey now.
My world is a better place for having you in it.
Love you roomie!

Thank you Yalina and Vanessa for being part of my tribe.
Big love to you both soul sisters.

To the rest of my friends and family.
Thank you for providing love, family dinners, thoughtful
heartfelt gifts and for babysitting.
Thank you for rallying around me with support, for every single
prayer and good vibe you sent my way. You pulled me through.
You are all friggen rock stars in my eyes.

Thank you to the AMAZING nurses at
Sister Caritas Cancer Center! Your smiling faces, compassionate
natures and deeply present hugs were like mother's milk on
treatment days. You were angels to me and for that I will be
forever grateful.

To my surgeon, gastroenterologist and oncologist; I am blessed
to know you. Even you Dr. M! Don't worry, I won't let the
other patients know you have a sense of humor or that you've
been known to crack a smile or two.

To Julie and Fred, thank you for constructive criticism and
encouraging me to develop my craft. Thank you for influencing
and inspiring me, for challenging and believing in my abilities as
a writer.

CONTENTS

FOREWORD
Early Loss, New Hope

"For death begins with life's first breath,
And life begins at touch of death."
~John Oxenham

From the moment we take our first breath, we begin a journey through life which inevitably leads to death. Throughout the course of our lives, it is my belief that we have the potential to live out many different lifetimes as our souls evolve and grow.

We let go of our childhood selves to become our teenage selves, shedding our teenage selves to step into adulthood. As each new phase of life is reached, we continuously release old expressions of who we think we are to become the more authentic versions of who we are actually meant to be.

Many of us tempt fate as teenagers, under the misconceived notion that death is ever elusive because, *of course,* we're going to live forever. These unnecessary risks become "rights" of passage, or at the very least, learning experiences.

At the age of seventeen, I survived a near fatal car crash on a pitch black backroad - miraculously without a single broken bone in my body. After falling asleep at the wheel, minutes from my parent's home, the front passenger's side of my sedan bounced off a tree and sent my car reeling across the road, smashing it into another tree. The second collision ricocheted my car across the blacktop, again, where it finally stopped, nose first, into a third and final tree. The final collision saved my life because, unbeknownst to me, there was a small river on the other side of it just below the road.

When my eyes finally opened after hitting the last tree, I screamed into the darkness for help. Uncontrollable sobs wailed from my chest as though I were grieving my own death. My left leg was pinned, in a bent position with my knee pressed up against the dashboard, between the steering wheel and the door. No matter how hard I fought to open that door, it wouldn't budge. The door finally gave way after what felt like hours of fighting against it, and I fell to the ground as it did. I couldn't put pressure on my left leg without being in a state of unbearable, excruciating pain. I pulled myself up slowly, putting as much weight on the good leg as I could. Eventually I was able to find my cell phone, call for help and was transported to the local hospital once the ambulance arrived.

The look of raw sadness in my mother's tear-filled eyes as she looked upon me when she got to the hospital, knowing I could have died, is something forever ingrained in my memory. A look of pain that would be revisited some ten years later, when I was diagnosed with Stage III Colon Cancer.

From a very young age, the fragility of life made itself known to me through the incarnation of loss and my own near death experiences. My mother's brother passed away at the age of thirty-three when I was nearly five-years-old. During the first five years of my life, though, he quickly became my favorite.

Uncle "Teddy" was witty, fun and wonderfully handsome in his flannel shirts. His use of quirky satire got under my grandmother's skin like no other. When we heard, "Knock it off Teddy!", my mom and I knew it was only a moment or two before he was back at it again. He constantly joked that he'd love to give my waist-length hair a "trim." "Only about eight or nine inches!" - he'd say with a devious smile, chasing after me, making scissor-cutting movements with his fingers.

As the years passed - so did aunts, uncles, grandparents, my great-grandmother, and two of my cousins. None of which prepared me for the greatest heartache of my teenage years. I was fifteen when my first love made the ultimate sacrifice to save his best friend's life. He was one of the most incredible human beings I've known; loving and loyal, kind and selfless. There wasn't a day I wanted to be alive during that first year without him. His death sent me into a six-month catatonic depression.

I felt him with me in spirit; sitting on the edge of my bed as I cried out for him to come back or standing behind me when I washed dishes at the kitchen sink. I heard his voice in my head cracking jokes, and saw his smile in my mind as he laughed at how funny he thought he was.

A few years later, another devastating blow to my heart hit when my best friend passed away at the age of twenty-two. We were inseparable. When I hurt, he did everything to make it better. When he joined the Army, I wrote to him daily. When he came home from training, it was like he never left. He was the closest thing I had to a brother, in the absence of my three older brothers who had all moved out to start families of their own.

Death conditioned me to accept loss as a part of life, turning abrasive discomfort into a type of emotional solvent. Stuff it down, suck it up, life goes on, time heals the pain.

That all changed the day my son, Dominic, was born. He came into this world five weeks and five days early; a whopping five pounds, five ounces. The nurse practitioner who delivered him said he would have been nearly ten pounds, had I gone full term. Dom spent five days in the Neo-Natal Intensive Care Unit and another seven days in the Continuing Care Nursery. He was three days old before I could hold him for the first time. From the moment I held his fragile, newborn body in my hands - love gushed from my heart to my eyes in the form of joyful tears.

For the first time in my life, I felt I had something - someone - worth fighting for, worth staying on this Earth for no matter how hard it got. He needed me as much as I needed him. Dominic saved me from me and, little did I know, he would be my saving grace time and time again.

Five years and two and a half months later, my daughter Izabella was born. The biggest worry during my pregnancy for her was, "How will I ever love another child as much as I love my son?" I was so worried that I would reject her, or love my son more or not feel as connected to her as I did to her brother. Yet Izzy's birth was a preview of the magic to come.

My labor was short but the contraction pain was STRONG. As the nurses prepped me for a Cesarean, they sang Greek wedding songs, which immediately put my heart at ease. The nurse practitioner joked as she pulled Izzy free from within my womb. "Don't worry Amber, I'll do all of the work for you!" - she said with both love and humor. I couldn't help but to laugh. There she was; my sweet Izabella, covered in vernix, sucking her thumb and I fell in love.

When my cancer journey began, it felt like I should have had a much stronger reaction to being diagnosed. Then again, experiencing so much loss early on in life conditioned me to be stronger than had I not. My initial thoughts were, *what do I do next to get through this? What if I don't make it?* Envisioning Dom and Izzy's future without me around to, physically, witness their milestones was disheartening beyond any diagnosis.

Not seeing the bashful look on Dom's face as he knocked on his prom date's door, not being there for Izzy's first school dance or driving test, never having another one of her "good morning hugs" or never seeing Dom kick a soccer ball across a field again - tore me up emotionally.

Those very same thoughts lent me strength. They forced me to rise up, embrace my inner warrior and then break my heart open to let the healing in. That was the moment I promised myself to never stop "fighting like a girl" - not for me, but for my babes. Those wonderful, crazy little humans were my saving grace and they continue to be every day.

Cancer itself isn't a gift I'd wish upon anyone. It strips away your health, your mental clarity. It breaks down your body. It chips away at your spirit. It has the power to uproot your life completely, to challenge even the closest of relationships with friends, family and lovers.

Yet there is also such capacity for life in the belly of the beast. You can let it break you down, or break you open. You can let it be a death sentence, or a catalyst to live an extraordinary life. You can become bitter, angry, resentful and live in fear - or you can turn to gratitude, shift to love and embrace everyday you're alive as a gift.

There are diseases and other types of cancer far worse than Colon Cancer. Even in terminal cases, you still have a choice in how you want your memory to live on. You still have the choice to prove everyone wrong and kick that cancer's ass all the way to recovery and remission. You *always* have the power of choice, *always*.

If you are sitting here now, reading a copy of this book, my hope in the chapters to come is that you realize there is greatness within *you*. It doesn't make me exceptional or extraordinary because I beat cancer. I went from being a broken-hearted, 118-pound cancer patient, living off of food stamps and public assistance, with no vehicle, unable to work, drowning in debt - to a financially self-sustaining, 140-pound, healthy, cancer free, life-loving, passion-pursuing, woman of worth.

If I found a way to heal my body, mind and spirit, to pursue what makes me feel passionate about waking up every morning - as a single mom, who comes from quite literally nothing - then why can't *you*? The answer is simple. You absolutely *can*. Everything you need for the journey, no matter how hard that road may be, is already within *you*. The power to overcome adversity lies within *us all*.
We need only to tap into it.

10

INTRODUCTION
Before Cancer

"Denial ain't just a river in Egypt."
~Mark Twain

Prior to the Fall of 2013, just months before my cancer diagnosis, I'd spent years changing majors; from nursing to radiology, to medical assisting then veterinary medicine. The passion to professionally pursue writing tugged on my heartstrings with fervor, the way a relentless child pulls their parent's sleeve toward the candy aisle.

Like any clueless, misled, twenty something does - I ignorantly swatted my creative muse away, not wanting to disappoint my family. After all, I had children of my own, on my own, to support. Going into the medical field offered a sense of security that, previous conditioning led me to believe, a writing career simply did not. I continued studying veterinary medicine at Holyoke Community College, completely going against my intuitive calling.

Perhaps, on a subconscious level, I intentionally failed the one veterinary course I so desperately needed to pass. Then again, maybe my soul decided to answer intuition's calling, knowing full well who I was destined to be – and let's face it, she wasn't rooting for *veterinary technician*. Either way, failing to pass Veterinary Anatomy and Physiology meant being cut loose from HCC's Veterinary Technician program. It comes as no surprise that I wasn't the least bit saddened by the college's requirement to do so.

Under the advice of one exceptionally witty and wise woman, Professor Kizershot, I finally heeded my heart's calling and changed my major to Creative Writing. The following Spring, I graduated with honors from HCC.

Before graduation I was guided by another wonderful (albeit persistent) mentor of mine, Professor Cooksey. In the top left corner of an assignment I turned in for class, he wrote: "Don't you want to take the practicum and write for the (campus) paper?" He had been asking for weeks prior to that but eventually his determination finally beat my stubborn rebellion.

Several articles later, as Features Editor of the campus paper, I enrolled at the University of Massachusetts, Amherst as a Journalism transfer student for the Fall of 2013.

Mid-June of 2013, I became Level I certified as a Reiki practitioner. My seven-year-old son, Dominic, excelled in sports during both the Spring and the Fall. My two-year-old daughter, Izzy, started gymnastics in September. Even my long-distance beau, Mark, was pretty amazing. The year felt so full of promise.

Toward the end of my Spring semester at HCC, in 2013, I felt more tired than usual. Ego brushed it aside, "I'm staying up too late for finals," I told myself. Plus, Izzy grew more mobile every day. Being a woman, raising a boy, was another animal altogether. Exhaustion itself wasn't a huge red flag when you considered my daily "hat change" between chauffeur, chef and housekeeper amongst other roles.

Then in June, I noticed a trivial amount of blood in my stool. It could have been anything; from stress or lack of sleep, maybe from something I ate? A week or so later it happened again. Within weeks it became a daily occurrence. Each time more blood was present in my stool, but never in the water of the toilet. No matter how much I slept, it didn't make a difference. My energy levels were next to null.
The bleeding got worse as weeks passed, intense pain plagued my abdomen. The pain ranged from sharp, radiating stabs to dull, throbbing pulses that confined me to the couch.

One particular morning the pain was excruciating. I was driving to UMass, with Mark on speaker phone in the car. About ten to fifteen minutes into our conversation, the pain started but I continued to drive. When he realized I was writhing in agony, from the cries I let out, he told me to pull the car over immediately.

Tears filled my eyes. My insides twisted as pins and needles clawed desperately at my organs, choked breath from my lungs and drowned logic from my mind. Mark stayed on the phone with me, calming me until I was able to turn the car around. It was the longest five-mile drive of my life. The pain dissipated within ten minutes of me arriving home.

A day or so later, my primary care doctor had me come into the office for an exam and ordered a full panel of bloodwork. The results came back normal. In a detrimental state of denial, I directed more attention toward my children and academic goals. I was "too young" at twenty-nine, "too healthy" and "too active" for it to be anything serious.

Besides, the tests were all normal right? It was stress or something in my diet, it would go away on its own. Diligence was my ego's middle name, in her determination to twist the intuitive truth. My parents, siblings and closest friends were oblivious to the warning signs my body was sending.

A new semester began in late August, early September of 2013 just months after my symptoms began, but I was ecstatic! I applied for the *Travel Writing in Sicily* course, immediately after the Fall semester began. If accepted, it meant spending ten days in sunny Sicily during Spring break 2014. Half of the class would put together a writing portfolio. The other half would create a photography portfolio, based on different assignments given throughout travel in Sicily.

There was no question for me, I *had* to go on this trip. It would be my first time out of the United States. Not only that, but it would give me an opportunity to reconnect with my Sicilian roots. Priceless in my eyes, no matter the cost of the trip.

As part of the application process, I had to answer the following question: "If you were trapped on a remote island somewhere and had only one song that you could listen to, what would it be?" I chose the song *I'm Alive* by Michael Franti and Spearhead.

My sister, Kimmy, introduced me to Michael Franti's music earlier that summer. It was one of those perfect family barbecue type of days; clear skies, burgers on the grill, our kiddos ran around the yard while my sis was a rock star of a hostess. In true Kim fashion, she made sure there were plenty of feel good vibes on the radio and everyone had enough to fill their plates. How poignantly ironic that, in the year to come, that song would be a constant source of strength as I fought for my life.

By October, my mother's growing concern caused her to routinely question the amount of sleep I was getting. I'd reply with, "stayed up late studying" or "kids fell asleep past bedtime," even on nights when it was the farthest thing from truth. In her gut, she knew I was full of shit when I told her I was fine. Moms are wonderful bullshit detectors, mine especially.

In early October, my body decided she was tired of being ignored. My mom had taken off for her usual 2:30 to 11 p.m. shift. Nothing seemed out of the ordinary. I was tired and there was still blood in my stool but nothing *else* was out of the ordinary.

Dom was already home from school, and Izzy from daycare, when it happened. Around 4pm I made sure they were contently distracted for the next hour so I could sit down and get some classwork done.

When I sat down at my roll top desk, an unexpected rumble roared from my belly, followed by obnoxiously loud gas. I paused for a moment and thought to myself "I just shit my pants." *(and no, you're not a terrible human being if you laughed when you read that)* I wasn't entirely sure I had shit my pants but I knew something wasn't right. I sat up enough to feel the back of my jungle-green capris to see if they were wet. When I pulled my hand away from checking the outside of the cotton fabric, it sent me reeling into the bathroom in a state of sheer and utter panic.

Blood.

My hand was covered in bright, red blood. There was so much it soaked straight through my pants and completely covered my palm and fingers.

When I ran into the bathroom I felt like I was going to vomit. You know when you feel like you're about to have the worst case of diarrhea you've ever had in your life? That's exactly how I felt. Except it wasn't watery stool coming out, it was blood. I flushed the toilet and washed my hands but quickly found my way to the porcelain throne again. More blood filled the toilet bowl.

Dom came to the bathroom door after he and Izzy heard me screaming and crying.

My head was spinning; what was happening? What was wrong with me? I couldn't breathe. I flushed the toilet again, washed my hands and ran out of the bathroom long enough to grab my cell phone. I ran back into the bathroom and called my Mom at work. She instantly headed home to take me to the emergency room.

We waited for nine hours in that emergency room. They checked my vital signs three times but I was never seen by a doctor. After nine hours of waiting in the ER, and seeing the sun come up, my mom and I decided to go home. By the time we got home, we had just a few short hours to rest before going in to see my primary care doctor. He wanted to do an in-house rectal exam to make sure it wasn't a hemorrhoid or ruptured vessel.

As lovely a family practitioner as he is, he didn't carry any type of specialty certification in the field of gastroenterology. In the core of my being I knew it wasn't something he could do anything about so I declined the exam. Only a specialist would be able to help me from here on out. My PCM ordered a full panel of bloodwork and sent a referral off to the insurance company for a gastroenterology visit. The results of those tests only fueled my stubbornness. Everything came back within normal range.

In the weeks spent waiting to see the GI specialist, my mother's worry only escalated. Her mind wasn't put at ease by the test results, as mine clearly had been. Within a week or two of my frantic episode, and subsequent ER visit, a dear friend and fellow Reiki practitioner reached out to me.

The only people who knew what was happening at this point were my parents, an aunt, an uncle and the guy I had been dating since June. My Reiki Practitioner friend - who we'll call "Buddha" - had no prior knowledge of my condition. She asked if I was interested in attending a Reiki share clinic at the center we'd both been certified at. It was way too long since we spent time catching up and even more time since I had attended a Reiki share. After confirming child care with my mom, Buddha and I made plans to meet the following Sunday night.

The night of the Reiki share, she arrived before me and was already waiting inside the building by the time I pulled into the driveway. I parked the car and made my way toward the entrance. My stomach gurgled and churned, my feet continued marching forward. Once inside, greetings were exchanged and we gathered into groups of three. Buddha and I were in the same group.

When it was my turn to receive Reiki, my stomach did somersaults and flip flops within my abdominal cavity. More gurgling noises bellowed out as my abdominal area soaked up healing like a sponge.

Once the session was over, we all mingled for a bit before my friend and I finally headed outside. Once we were near our vehicles, away from the building, she gave me a deep look of empathetic concern and asked, "What the hell is going on with your stomach woman?" She shared how hot her hands were during my session, how she kept being drawn to send Reiki to my abdominal area. I told her everything and promised to keep her in the loop, and she promised to keep me in her prayers.

About two weeks after the Reiki share clinic and three weeks after I first hemorrhaged, I finally met with "Dr. S" the Gastroenterologist, on Halloween of all days. The morning filled my mind with anxious thoughts about what could possibly be wrong. My mom and I drove in together, parked the car and made our way to the office building. Not a word was exchanged. We walked together with worry and anxiety, as we contemplated infinite possibilities - none of which seemed realistically optimistic. After checking in at the front desk, with heavy hearts, we patiently waited until I was called in by the medical assistant.

My mom looked to me for approval. Would it be okay if she wanted to come in? She didn't say it out loud but I knew her well enough to know that's exactly what she was thinking. I asked her if she was coming in with me and she eagerly jumped up like a mama kangaroo ready to run miles in the outback to save her baby joey. The medical assistant took my vitals and as quickly as she led us into the room, she said the doctor would be in shortly and let herself out.

When Dr. S walked into the room her empathetic compassion put my mind at ease. Between her beaming, bubbly personality and comical bedside manner - I knew I was in good hands. She was hopeful my condition was something minor and treatable, but thought it prudent to schedule a colonoscopy as a precautionary measure.

How could she have thought otherwise? Aside from extreme fatigue and irregular bleeding, I hadn't lost any weight and I wasn't in chronic pain. About a week later, though, I *was* in pain. Excruciating abdominal pain, just above my navel. Dr. S's office scheduled me in for a same-day-sick-appointment. The physician's assistant ordered blood work and a CT scan with IV contrast. The test results, once again, came back unremarkable. My appendix was slightly inflamed but the doctor didn't believe it was cause for concern.

Yet, something felt off to *me*. I knew my body, and I was ready to admit that something wasn't right.

MY CANCER DIARY

1

DECEMBER 2013
Into the Chrysalis

"We must never forget the importance of gratitude. Say thank you when your heart is full and when it breaks, and when you are alone and sad, and when you dance with joy, and when things are lost and found again. Day and night, give thanks for this incredibly beautiful, tragic gift called life."
~author unknown

Friday - December 20, 2013

Today was *the day*. My first colonoscopy. Everything was a blur around me when Dr. S was going over the results with Mom. My mom was crying, sobbing uncontrollably. I was on my left side in the hospital bed, my right hand clutched to the bed rail, left hand tucked under my side after the procedure.

When I heard my mom crying, I rolled over in her direction. There were nurses in the recovery room, faces solemn with worry. One was wiping tears from her face but suddenly looked away when she noticed me waking up. I turned over to feel an icy hand take mine. My mom wiped her own tears away as she wrapped her fingers around my hand.

Slowly, I drifted back into consciousness. Dr. S spoke with my mom. Her words were heavy but didn't register. "I'm so sorry. It doesn't look good. We have to wait on the biopsy to come back but from my experience, it looks like cancer." There was talk of polyps and surgery to remove a malignant tumor from my colon when I felt Mom give my hand a sympathetic rub. Without a spoken word, I knew what she was telling me. "I'm here with you sweetheart. We're going to get through this. You're going to be okay, we can do this."

Turns out the tumor is roughly four centimeters in diameter and located in my sigmoid colon. There were polyps too but Dr. S removed them to be biopsied. She's fairly certain it's colon cancer. Hot tears rushed down my cheeks when I asked her if the surgery could be done before March but I don't remember feeling much of anything in that moment. I just remember thinking *I have to go to Sicily*.

Today's findings didn't surprise me. My body has been sending signals for months now that something was wrong. I was just too damn stubborn to listen.

Everything was a blur on the car ride home. Dom and Izzy are with relatives right now so the house is pretty quiet. Too quiet, somber even.

Mom doesn't know it but I can hear her crying, from my room, out in the kitchen. She's talking to Auntie about the results. I want to comfort her. I want to tell her how strong I am, that we'll get through this together. I hate seeing her like this, she's gone through so much already in her life…now this. I want to be there for her but I can't.

I don't feel sad or angry or depressed. I don't feel anything. Am I supposed to feel *nothing?* Shouldn't there at least be a feeling of disappointment? You would think I'd be wondering "how could this happen to me?" or "why me?" but I'm not. Cancer doesn't give a shit about age or any of that bullshit. *So why not me?* The only thing I feel is emptiness, I'm totally numb.

Sunday - December 22, 2013

I'm so angry with so many things in my life lately. I believe in the power of thought manifesting into reality, but also the power of gratitude. Which means that whether or not I want to admit it, I drew everything I'm angry about into my life. Through action or inaction and every decision I have ever made, this is all my own doing. I've put on a mask of superficial happiness for so long but, in reality, the pain is still there. I swear to God, all of these suppressed fucking issues are why my body manifested cancer.

So much anger. Resentment. Anger with others for treating me harshly, anger with myself for never taking a stand against it. Issues I've yet to resolve within myself. The bullying throughout junior high; classmates writing insidiously cruel things about me in yearbooks, an upper classman slamming me into a locker threatening to beat me up. Countless other incidents. The bullying went on for years before I finally stood up for myself.

Even now, at 29, I don't feel *good enough* to be in a healthy, loving relationship. Clearly, judging by my previously unhealthy relationship patterns. Deep down, I know I don't love myself. I'll never be genuinely happy with anyone else until I'm happy with myself.

Yet, things have been wonderful with Mark. He flew me out to California a few weeks ago, my first visit to the West Coast. It was beautiful. I marveled over how ocean air didn't hit my nose with the pungent, welcoming smell of baked seaweed as it does here on the East Coast. In California, at least near the Santa Monica Pier, the smell of ocean lingered close to shore. It didn't hit my nostrils until I was ankle deep in the waves.

Mark is kind, thoughtful, attentive to my needs, encourages me to be my best self. I don't want to bring him into the Pandora's box of suppressed emotions cancer just opened up for me. I won't do that to him, he deserves so much more. I felt nothing a few days ago after my colonoscopy but now there's only anger. Deep, seething, fiery anger. It's too much for anyone to take on.

What I want more than anything is a place of my own, to finish my degree and have a career that I'm passionately in love with. It's exactly what I was working on when I was diagnosed. Only three semesters left until graduation, until the possibility of moving anywhere in the country and having total independence again became a reality. All of that is on hold now, because I'll need major surgery and possibly chemotherapy.

My mom and I were told that "Colon cancer is one of the better cancers to have, as long as it's caught early on." I'm grateful my cancer is treatable and has a high prognosis for being cured but the doctors should probably work on their delivery of that information. *Better* cancer? Clearly they've never been cancer patients. When you're on the receiving end of a cancer diagnosis, there is no such thing as a "better cancer." I'm just so fucking angry today. I had so much going for me. A cancer diagnosis was the last thing I needed.

Everything is happening so fast now. A surgical consultation has been scheduled for me, Christmas Eve of all days. According to cancer.org, Colon Cancer is the second leading cause of cancer death in men and women combined??? But I've got the "better cancer" according to my doctors, so I'll just go ahead and *relax* then. Right. I'm supposed to go to Sicily in March. I don't know how all of this is going to affect things.

Tuesday - December 24, 2013

I'm feeling completely overwhelmed after meeting with the surgeon, Dr. M. He ran through everything with lightning speed like a grocery store checklist. *Milk, bread, eggs, we're going to remove eight to nine inches of your colon, there's a possibility of infection, these are the statistics and probability of what can go wrong, peanut butter, cereal, oatmeal, you should be fine though since I've performed hundreds of these surgeries before.*

Surgery on New Year's Eve. Removal of part of my colon, part of my rectum too. He doesn't feel I'll need a colostomy bag but nothing is for certain until he has a look inside.

His words forever engrained in my memory; "You're pretty fortunate, you know, tumors like this don't usually bleed. If you would have waited another six months, there would have been nothing we could do for you."

Six months. That's twenty-six weeks. Roughly 182 days and I would have been terminal. I'm feeling numb again.

Thursday - December 26, 2013

*"Wake at dawn with a winged heart and give thanks for
another day of living."*
~Kahlil Gibran

This year, me and the kids spent Christmas
with my sister, Kim, and her hubby's side of the
family. I've been feeling so angry since my
colonoscopy, so wrapped up in my own misery that I
was losing sight of what still matters. So many things
were planned for my future until less than a week ago.
Everything was falling into place, finally. Then came
the cancer diagnosis and my power was completely
ripped away. Any sense of order or control, gone.

The uncertainty that crept in, replaced any
hope I had left. It was getting to be more than I can
handle. I shut down. Numbed myself to the pain of
loss that accompanied not having certainty over my
future. Then I got angry, really fucking angry. How
dare this happen to me and ruin my plans for the
future! Then I stayed angry. Not so good for my
health, I'm sure.

Spending time with Kim and my nieces and
her husband's side of the family took me back to
gratitude, to that place of having faith that all is as it
should be. *La famiglia è tutto*, the family is everything
and they've given me new hope. The presence of love

all around me was true, spiritual, soul-medicine. It permeated my senses, dismantled personal grief and brought me to a sacred space of inner peace. I know intuitively, now, everything will be alright.

Good old "Saint Patrick" gave me a coin with St. Jude, patron saint of desperate causes, on it and mala prayer beads as well as a little statue of Buddha…the actual Buddha, not a statue of my other friend who I lovingly call Buddha. My new gifts are like personal talismans, here to lend me a bit of strength when I start losing faith again. There's a long road ahead of me but I'm going to get through this. I don't know how, but I know I will.

Saturday - December 28, 2013

My passport came in today! I was out and about running errands when I found a lucky penny with my birth year on it. Things are looking up!

Monday - December 30, 2013

"You will never have this day with your children again. Tomorrow they'll be a little older than they were today. Today is a gift. Just breathe, notice, study their faces and little feet. Pay attention. Relish the charms of the present. Enjoy today. It will be over before you know it."
~Jen Hatmaker

Getting as many hugs and snuggles from my munchkins as I can today. Izzy is heading to Kimmy's house for the next week. Dom will be with my parents and then I think Kimmy's too, or something like that. Either way, I won't be seeing either of my babes for the next week while I undergo surgery and recover in the hospital.

They don't know I have cancer or why I'm going to the hospital. Izzy is so young. She wouldn't understand even if I told her. All she knows is that she gets to have a week long slumber party at Auntie Kimmy's house with cousins…and that she doesn't get to have "milkies" anymore.

Dr. M told me it's a good time to stop nursing Izzy since I may need chemo and/or radiation and I won't be able to once I have surgery. I believe his exact words were; "How old is your daughter? Two and a half? Yeah, it's probably time to stop nursing her anyhow." *(Present day note, Dr. M turns out to be way less of a dick than he sounds and is one of my absolute favorite humans.)*

Dom, though, he's older and sharp as a tac for his age. He knows Mom is sick and the doctors have to take the sickness out of my body but he doesn't know it's cancer. I haven't thought about how to tell him or *if* I should tell him at all.

I've decided to wait until after surgery to tell him anything else. The doctors won't know until then if I need further treatment. Best not to unnecessarily worry him or stress myself out about telling him. Not until I know for sure what's going to happen next.

Tuesday - December 31, 2013
weight: 118 pounds/53.52 kilograms

Today is the day, 2013. You threw me for a loop but I have an exceptionally supportive family by my side. I'm scared about this surgery but Mom and Dad are here with me. On January 1, I'm waking up healthier than I've ever been.

2
JANUARY 2014
Have Faith

*"We must be willing to let go of the life we have planned,
so as to have the life that is waiting for us."*
~Joseph Campbell

Wednesday - January 1, 2014

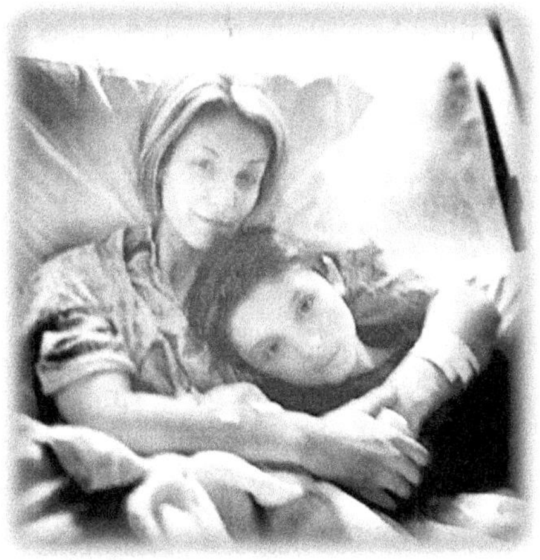

Mom and Dad stopped by today with Dom. It was so good to see them. I didn't know how Dom would take it or if he should even come by. At one point my parents walked out to give me and Dom some time alone. We were talking about how he's been during my hospital stay when he suddenly became quiet. His face started to turn red around his eyes, like it does when he's upset. He wouldn't look at me but I could see the tears welling up in his eyes; "Are you going to die Mom?"

A stream of tears raced down my cheeks. I brushed them away hoping Dom didn't see me deeply saddened by his question. As much as I'd sworn to myself that I'm going to fight this cancer with all I've got, I don't know for certain what the future holds.

I looked him in the eyes and said, with great conviction, "I'm not going anywhere kiddo." God, I hope I'm right.

Friday - January 3, 2014

Had the most miraculous experience after surgery Tuesday night. Woke up in the middle of the night, in intense pain, so I prayed hard, asking the angels to be with me. I started doing a self-Reiki session when I felt what I can only describe as the divine presence of God by my side.

I was physically alone in that room. No doctors, nurses or family members were present. There's no rational, logical reason to explain why it felt like there was a legion of support rallying around me. Yet I know I wasn't truly alone. I closed my eyes and continued the Reiki session. Calm, peace and love washed over me.

By Wednesday night, within 24 hours of doing Reiki, my severe pain was gone. I know some people don't believe in all that "hooey" as Dom likes to call it, but I sure do. One of my friends made a joke about it, telling me "They must have given you some pretty good pain meds!" We laughed about it, especially considering he's an atheist and I'm deeply spiritual, but in my heart I know there were angels by my side that night.

By the way, Dr. M said I can go home today, a whole day earlier than anticipated. YES! He walked in just as I finished washing my hair in the bathroom sink. There's no way I could take another day without at least washing my hair. He came in to tell me I can go home…and oh yeah, I can take that long overdue shower (my words, not his, although I'm sure he would have agreed). At least my hair is washed. I'm still on a liquid diet but I finally pooped since Tuesday's surgery so there's a bonus.

He said I'm making a speedy recovery. Checked in for surgery Tuesday afternoon and haven't needed heavy pain meds since Wednesday. Just ibuprofen here and there. Pretty sure I've willed away the pain because I couldn't deal with how the meds made me feel.

After eight Heparin shots, seven intravenous lines (including two that were blown) and three early morning wake up calls by phlebotomists – it feels euphoric to know I'll be sleeping in my own bed tonight. I miss my kids. I miss my allergy prone dog. I miss the comfort of being wrapped up in my favorite blanket.

It brings me to tears when I think about all of the wonderful people praying for me, wishing me well. I couldn't do this without them. The outpour of love and support has been unbelievable.

Saturday - January 4, 2014

Animals are so intuitive. My seventy-pound Shepherd mix, Bella, has always been a jumper and a hugger but not much of a snuggler. Since I've come home from the hospital she looks at me with these sad eyes and keeps her ears down while wagging her tail. Like she knows I'm too fragile to jump on right now.

When I pat my hand on my leg - letting her know it's okay to approach - she cautiously runs over, body low to the ground, shaking her furry booty the whole way, as if to say "Yes! She's okay! I get my back scratched by Mom again!" God, it feels so good to be home. Thank you for these moments.

Sunday - January 5, 2014

To the powers that be, thank you for all the strength. Now if you could just send me some patience, it would be much appreciated.

Wednesday - January 8, 2014

Trying to take it easy today, still recovering from major surgery. I guess depending on how many lymph nodes come back as cancerous, if any, the doctors will know what steps to take next. Haven't heard back yet from the surgeon's office but hopefully I'm cancer free!

Today I organized Dom's books, did the dishes, made homemade organic chicken noodle soup and I'm officially wiped out. My stomach muscles are achy. I'm a tad bit sore when I stand up to move around but I managed to get through grocery shopping plus a quick stop at Target. I'm not

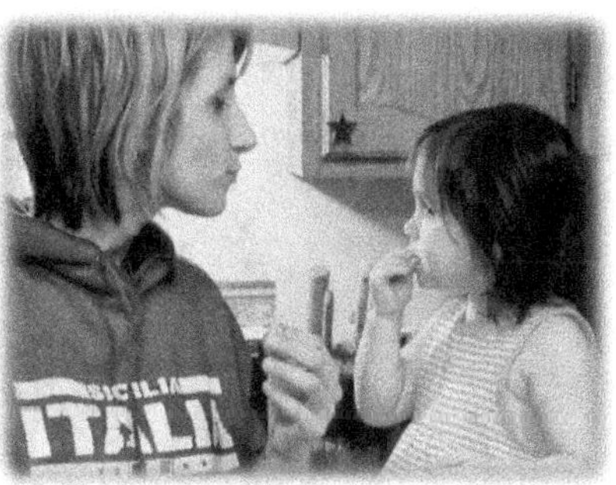

allowed to drive until Dr. M gives the "OK" so Mom has been my personal chauffeur for the day.
Izzy was hugging me tonight after her bath. When her damp hair touched my nose, tears flooded down my cheeks. The smell of coconut shampoo as she hugged me was emotionally overpowering.

I'm trying to be strong for her, for Dom, for my parents, for everyone really. Which means I can't feel how hard it is to raise two kids on my own while going through chemo. If I allow myself to feel the pain, it's going to break me down and that would break the hearts of everyone around me.

The thought of not being here to see Dom and Iz off to prom, or watch them walk across the stage at graduation, not riding shotgun during their driving lessons or being absent for soccer games, not tucking them in at night - it's more than I can handle right now. I'm not strong enough, yet, to let *that* kind of pain in.

Speaking of strength, Sunday was a trying day with Dom. He's processing so much with me being sick. He knows that something is wrong with Mom, but I haven't told him yet

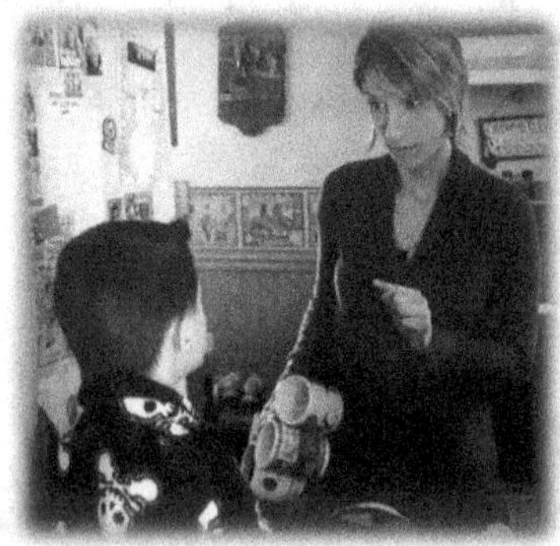

that it's cancer. I don't know how to have that conversation with him or what to say without him thinking he's going to lose me. Truth is, I don't know what's going to happen yet. It's best to wait and see what the results are of the biopsy and go from there. Whether I need chemo and radiation is yet to be determined.

I should be getting more rest today. It's much needed after Izzy, the gymnast, accidentally kicked me a few times in the stomach.

She was so funny today. I overheard her telling Mom, "I swear to God Grandma! You got one more! That's it! No more, you go away!" I'm not even sure what she was talking about but whatever it was, she meant business!

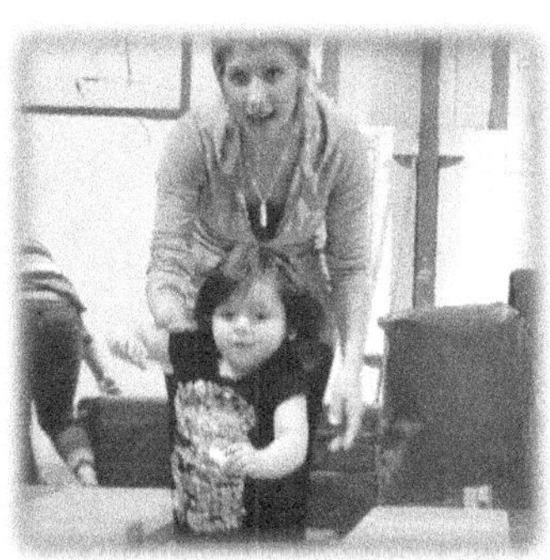

* * *

Thursday - January 9, 2014

Received word today from Dr. M about the biopsies sent out after New Year's Eve's surgery. Three of my lymph nodes tested positive for cancer. It's infiltrated the lymphatic tissue, my sigmoid colon and rectum. I've become a candidate for chemo and radiation and I've officially been diagnosed with Stage III Colon Cancer.

He was asking if I've thought about conceiving more children, explaining that infertility - amongst other things - was a possible side effect. Hearing the word "infertility" left a pit of despair in my belly; as my femininity, power and strength were all ripped away at once. It's going to take a few days to process this.

Friday - January 10, 2014

Feeling thankful for all of my friends and family. For their prayers, love, support and positive energy. It's saddened them knowing I'll have to go through chemo and radiation. But I'm still here, still fighting. I've got every intention of being around for many years to come. This is another hurdle to overcome, test of strength and will. This is just the beginning.

On another note, Izzy let out a whole hearted chuckle in her sleep last night. Those moments are the ones that keep me going. I don't want to miss a single one.

Sunday - January 12, 2014

I've been working on shifting toward gratitude since my conversation with Dr. M a few days ago. I've thought about my close girlfriends and their journeys with infertility, their pain and perseverance through years of being told they wouldn't be able to conceive. Yet they were mamas now to beautiful, healthy children.

My thoughts turned toward my own two blessings. I thought about how close I was to losing Dom so many times. Twelve weeks into my pregnancy, I was put on bed rest because I began to miscarry. Dom made it to 34 weeks' gestation when my contractions started. They came on sharp and fast. We made it to the hospital just in time. They told me he was in fetal distress and his heart rate quickly dropped. Nurses and doctors prepared me for an emergency Cesarean and, nearly six weeks before his due date, Dominic was born.

It would be another three days before I held him because of all the tubes and wires connected to him within the warmth of his incubator. He spent the first week of his life in the Neonatal Intensive Care Unit and the second week in a Continuing Care Nursery.

I thought about my daily visits, sometimes several times a day. Thought about when I came home from the hospital without him. My parents and Felipe marveled over how well composed I was, until I walked into the nursery. Two steps in, that's all it took. I fell to the ground and cried and cried. Eventually he came home, and now he's 8-years-old.

There were lots of little bumps in the beginning with Dom; jaundice, colic, bronchiolitis, tubes in his ears, adenoids and tonsils removed, an asthma diagnosis. I'd go through it all again, a million times over, to be his mother. To be present for every open house, parent teacher conference, for every lesson learned, for every tantrum. All of it is such a gift.

That's what I've been focusing on these past few days. Gratitude for my children. How could I be so selfishly distraught over the possibility of not having children when there were countless women out there who longed to hold a child of their own, or their own child once more? When I stopped focusing on children I may never have after treatment, and focused more on the two beautiful babes in front of me, infertility didn't matter anymore.

Without Dom and Izzy; there'd be no fight within me, no desire to become the best version of me I can, no strength to carry on. I would have surrendered a long time ago and let God take me *home* if it weren't for those crazy knuckleheads. Gratitude is helping me realize our family *is* complete.

Also, only two months until Spring break in Italy! Passport is all set. Sandy beaches of Sicily, fine wine and olive oil - I'm there already. Something to most definitely look forward to.

Monday - January 13, 2014

There are 86,400 seconds in a day according to my calculator, if I calculated correctly. I plan on using at least a few of them to give thanks for all I have; air, breath and lungs, clothes on my back, healthy food to eat, Dom and Izzy's smiles, friendships. Replacing every possible complaint with a few words of gratitude.

Tuesday - January 14, 2014

Dr. M told me he spoke with the radiologist. She let him know radiation therapy would be of marginal gain to me. Given my age, long-term risk far outweighs the benefits. The medical team has decided to cancel radiation altogether. (thank you God!)
I have to meet with an oncologist next week. Chemotherapy is still part of the treatment plan but I'm undeniably elated that radiation has been taken out of treatment plans.

My older brother, Nate, has started calling me "Superwoman." I find this slightly ironic since all I ever wanted to be when I grew up was a superhero. While all of my friends were playing pretend with Barbie and princess castles, I was obsessed with pretending to be Storm and Rogue from *Marvel's X-Men.*
Storm was a force to be reckoned with, she didn't take shit from anyone.

When I discovered *Teenage Mutant Ninja Turtles* I wanted to be as defiantly independent as April O'Neil. Although if someone asked my mom, I'm sure she'd tell them I had it down to an art before I ever started watching four butt-kicking, pizza-eating, "heroes in a half shell."

Wednesday - January 15, 2014

Dom's God-mom has got me hooked on juicing! She's been so supportive. Thankful for her. Picked up apples, oranges, limes and kale…
Later that day…
Note to self, juicing requires A LOT of fruit and veggies and doesn't yield much juice. Cleaning the processor is a pain but honestly it's worth every drop! I've been juicing for most of the day, it's *that* good.

Thursday - January 16, 2014

Steri-strips from abdominal surgery are starting to fall off. Cleaning out the basement, kiddos entertaining themselves. Me and Dom's song comes on the radio, *(You Make Me Feel Like) A Natural Woman*, by Aretha Franklin. He stops what he's doing to look over at me.

Took everything in me not to cry in that moment. My life was blessed the day that munchkin was born. He may be a royal handful some days but Dom has helped me become a better woman. I'm that much stronger for raising him.

Wednesday - January 22, 2014
weight: 124.2 pounds / 56.33 kilograms

"Faith is taking the first step, even when you don't see the whole staircase."
-Dr. Martin Luther King Jr.

Today's office visit with my new oncologist, Dr. Roes, left so many unanswered questions in my mind. His words spun my thoughts around like a ballerina performing endless pirouettes. Thankfully Uncle D accompanied me. I imagined him as the fixed focal point, a presence to keep me centered while my internal world held on for dear life. Auntie, his wife, would have been there with us too but she came down with something last night.

I was given a six-page packet about chemotherapy side effects to read when I got home. Seriously, that many pages in eight-point font? My knowledgeable oncologist had overlooked the fact that I'm a full-time student, single mother of two, chauffeur for after school and weekend activities, home chef, laundry connoisseur and all around busy woman.

Info packets are great for childhood vaccines or what type of pet insurance you need to purchase, even cancer diagnosis, but not for an initial consult. This was the person who held my fate in their hands for the next six months. All sense of control was being handed over to him in regard to my health.

I needed him to go over everything with me, in detail. I needed a practitioner who held the intention of being present in the moment. What I needed to hear was, "*I'm here for you with any questions, whatever you need. We're going to get you through this.*"

Instead what I got was more or less, "*Twenty-nine-year-old female, presented with malignant adenocarcinoma of the colon. Here's how we're going to treat your illness and in six months you'll be good as new! See ya!*" Those weren't his words exactly, but close enough. As quickly as he came into the room, he was gone. I felt like someone sold me a lemon at a used car dealership.

Thursday - January 23, 2014

"I believe in the person I want to become."
~Anonymous

Next week I go in for day surgery to have a Porta Cath placed under my skin. It's an implant they'll place in the upper, left, area of my chest – just below my clavicle - that has a tube going directly into one of my veins. It's supposed to make receiving chemotherapy *easier*. Instead of the nurses needing to start a brand new intravenous line each chemo session, they can access my vein through the port.

I've been told that every two weeks, before chemo, I'll need to have bloodwork drawn as well. The *medicine* they're giving me is called FOLFOX-6. It stands for Leucovorin Calcium (Folinic Acid), Fluorouracil and Oxaliplatin.

Just in case I didn't have enough on my mind, I read the packet Dr. Roes sent home with me. The following is a list of some side effects it says FOLFOX causes. There are well over three dozen but these are the ones that stood out the most; abnormal heartbeat which may cause fainting, discomfort from light, confusion, dizziness, numbness, tingling, the sensation of pins and needles in your hands and feet, extreme sensitivity to cold temperatures (anything below room temperature), bleeding, diarrhea, vomiting, constipation, fatigue, increased risk of sunburn…the list continues on.

When I started reading the packet I thought to myself, *I should have gotten a second opinion. I don't want to do this.* I thought about holistic treatments and going to Dana Farber in Boston. I thought about not going through with chemotherapy and taking herbs and natural remedies to keep the cancer from coming back.

I know if I do all of those things, instead of chemo, Mom is going to worry herself sick. She's always been the worrier of the family and I know she'd be constantly over my shoulder, giving me *that look*, wondering if my cancer will come back, worrying she'll lose her daughter.

When I received the call about chemotherapy becoming part of the treatment regime, Mom was with me and she broke down crying. *I comforted her.*

That's what cancer does. It's not knowing you've been diagnosed with cancer or even knowing you have to be injected with completely toxic chemicals that kills your spirit. It's seeing what cancer does to everyone else around you that tears you up inside.

About a week or two after the Porta Cath is placed, I begin a six-month journey through bi-weekly chemo treatments. Time to suck it up and *fight like a girl.*

Saturday - January 25, 2014

"Repeat after me; I am stronger than this challenge,
this challenge is making me even stronger."
~unknown

It's taken me a day or two to get my bearings but I'm back to normal after meeting with the oncologist. Once I started thinking logically, I had a different mindset; *read the packet, this is your health, your body, your life. Highlight, underline anything you have questions about. On a separate sheet of note paper, write down your questions, your concerns. Take back your power from fear of the unknown.*

Everyone handles what life throws at them differently. Some people choose to let circumstance define them. I won't deny the role cancer currently plays in my life but I refuse to let it define me. Woman, mother, spiritual being, daughter, friend. These roles define the core of who I am; nurturer, kindness practitioner, lover, fighter, creator.

Life is a precious gift from the Universe. I will continue to live mine full of optimism, laughter, positive energy, gratitude and love...every...single...day. Cancer won't stop me from letting my light shine. If anything, cancer is going to amplify it.

Wednesday - January 29, 2014

Considering dropping one of my two morning classes but am most definitely keeping the two night ones. I must have been slightly crazy to think I could take on 13 credits, two kiddos and chemo all at once.

Thursday - January 30, 2014

One of my mom's friends shared this video with me on Facebook today. It was a Ted Talk by Dr. William Li, *Can we eat to starve cancer?* It was captivating.

Li discussed how abnormal angiogenesis (the development of new blood vessels) can cause cancer, as well as other diseases. He said, "Angiogenesis is the hallmark of cancer," and "all cancers start out microscopic, about the tip of a ballpoint pen, but without a blood supply providing oxygen and nutrients - they can't grow any larger."

At this point in the Ted Talk, my mind was blown. *Okay Dr. Li*, I thought to myself, *tell me how to prevent a blood supply from getting to those cancer cells*. I kept watching. He spoke of a relatively new therapy, called "Anti-angiogenic therapy." By selectively targeting the blood vessels that feed cancer cells, angiogenesis is blocked. It's different than traditional chemotherapy because it doesn't target our healthy cells like chemo does.

When Dr. Li showed before and after photos from both human and animal trials, the implications astounded me. A man's brain tumor was shrunk down to nearly nothing after four weeks of antiangiogenic therapy. A woman diagnosed with breast cancer, was treated for a tumor in one of her breasts. Within 4 weeks of taking Avastin (an anti-angiogenic agent), the tumor disappeared.

In animals, anti-angiogenic therapy produced the same results. An elderly *Boxer* with a tumor larger than a baseball underwent anti-angiogenic treatment and within 7 weeks, his tumor was gone. The same held true for a 20-year-old dolphin with squamous cell cancer of the mouth. Dr. Li continued; over the course of six-month, anti-angiogenic therapy, a horse diagnosed with a deadly form of cancer was in full remission.

Another part of his talk referenced specific foods, beverages and herbs acting as "natural angiogenic inhibitors." Basically, they're mother nature's ass-kicking cancer remedies. Resveratrol found in grapes and red wine, and Ellagic acid found in strawberries can both potently inhibit angiogenesis according to Dr. Li. He listed several foods his team is in the process of studying because of their anti-angiogenic properties; grapes, green tea, turmeric, cherries, earl grey, artichokes, grape seed oil, tomato, pumpkin, lavender. That's not even half the list.

I've already had major surgery; tumor removal, a third of my rectum taken out and eight or nine inches of my colon removed. Would the doctors consider anti-angiogenic therapy for me? Would the insurance cover it? Do I even bother at this point or do I just go through with chemo? What if I go on anti-angiogenic therapy and it doesn't work? Even with science backing it up, I'd be lying if I said I wasn't afraid of trying something unconventional with my health on the line. So much to take into consideration.

Friday - January 31, 2014

My brother Aaron and his wife Ragan drove up to visit me from Florida this week, their three kids in tow. I really *really* needed them today. Dom and Izzy's dad, Felipe, moved back in with us a few days ago. Today, I made him leave…for good.

3

FEBRUARY 2014
The Journey Begins

"Be thankful for every heartbreak, for they were planned. They come into your life just to reveal another layer of yourself to you, and then leave. Their purpose it to shake you up, tear apart your ego a little bit, show you your obstacles and addictions, break your heart open so new light can get in, make you so desperate and out of control that you have to transform your life and you do."
~unknown

Tuesday - February 4, 2014

I've got quite a bit of homework to do but I'm in desperate need of venting. I'm so angry with myself for letting Felipe move back in last week, only to kick him out again four days later.

We were together for so long, created two incredible lives together, married five and a half years, together for nearly a decade. For fifteen months I prayed for him during his deployment in Iraq, wrote to him daily, sent care packages in hopes of uplifting his spirits, reminding him that I was still going to be there for him when he came home. When deployment ended, the reality of our lives returning to "normal" set in.

Easy to love someone from a distance when you know deep down you're a toxic combination. Space and distance create a void filled by happy memories and the love you share, erasing pain and heartache from memory.

When Felipe returned from deployment, the grand illusion of how "beautifully different" life would be, was quickly shattered by the dysfunction of us. Long before deployment; slamming doors, thrown objects, abusive verbal put downs were a constant of our relationship. It only worsened when he came home.

We were both guilty of wanting to be right more than we wanted to make our marriage work. When it was good, I couldn't have imagined being with anyone else. But when it was bad, there were days I didn't want to get out of bed, or eat, or exist.

My son's Godmother, one of my dearest friends, once told me in reference to me and Felipe's marriage; "There's *too much* passion, sweetie, not enough logic." She was right, when your love is so intense that it borders obsession, you don't think half the time. You act impulsively based on emotion; jealousy and envy being the dominant ones. We were so young then, neither one of us knew how to be in a healthy relationship.

Years later, my mother recounted her own disheartening observation. She told me, "Do you remember when I flew out to Colorado to see you and help you out with Dom?" *(my son had undergone surgery to remove his tonsils and adenoids and tubes were placed in his ears during Felipe's deployment)* "When I saw you standing there, waiting for me in the terminal, it broke my heart to see you like that. You were so underweight and the twinkle in your eye was completely gone. You've always had this light about you since you were a little girl, but when I saw you, it's like my little Amber wasn't there anymore." Thinking back to how depressed I was, how disempowered I felt makes me tearful even now.

Dominic was my only saving grace. Many times the thought of ending my suffering, through irreversible means, came to mind. Each time, though, my heart turned to thoughts of Dominic. I thought of our Sunday picnics at *Garden of the Gods*, park trips to neighboring landmarks and local playground visits. I heard his raspy little voice, in my head, asking for apple juice or something to eat. His unconditional love saved me from my ego's ugly whispers. Time and time again he saved my life.

In spite of all that, somehow, I took Felipe back. I wonder if I was truly capable of being happy with him. So much has changed since the days when we'd have a heated argument and "split up" only to get back together ad nauseam.

I couldn't deny the fact that he'd been so kind since I was diagnosed with cancer. He'd call me after work on the way home to check in, made sure our kiddos were okay as well. He called everyday while I was in the hospital after surgery. He seemed undeniably different, like he was finally stepping into the potential of the man I knew he could be.

I've broken my heart, yet again, by falling for his potential. This is *finally* goodbye. It has to be. There's no other way.

I can forgive him in time, love him for being the man who graced me with the gift of Motherhood. Holding that space of love for him doesn't mean we should be together, doesn't warrant the right to be a part of my life in an intimate way. In the four days Felipe was here, he showed me that though many things have changed - his behavior toward me has not.

One week from today I'll be sitting in a chair for hours, feeling God knows what, on the receiving end of a chemical cocktail. I have to go through this alone now. Felipe won't be there to take Dom to practice when I'm too sick to get out of bed. He won't be there to tell me I'm still beautiful when my hair falls out. I'll sleep alone when I'm resting and won't have a partner to share this journey with. No one to kiss away my tears on the bad days or laugh with me on the good days. No one to look me in my eyes and say "Babe, I've got you, we'll get through this together." I feel so alone. How can I navigate through the rough sea ahead when I've lost my first mate?

The potential of who he could be to me during treatment, would be all those things and more. The reality is that his presence in my life during treatment would be to the detriment of my healing, on all levels.

I need to go to Sicily more than ever now. In the midst of this exhaustion and emotional fatigue, my soul is crying out for replenishment - spiritual sustenance.

My dreams are beginning to fizzle, I'm in desperate need of new hope.

Thursday - February 6, 2014

Today an incredibly significant piece of artwork was added to the living canvas of my body. It commemorates the most challenging battle I've faced yet, inspired by my recent diagnosis of colon cancer.

A navy blue colon cancer awareness ribbon is wrapped around the middle of a blue Morpho butterfly, with the words "fight like a girl" beneath it. It's symbolic of the extraordinary transformation cancer is taking me through and the decision to stand strong, whatever the journey brings.

When I was first diagnosed, I did so much research online. I wanted to know statistics, data, treatments, alternative therapy, holistic approaches, survival rate, support group info, the best oncologist, the best surgeon.

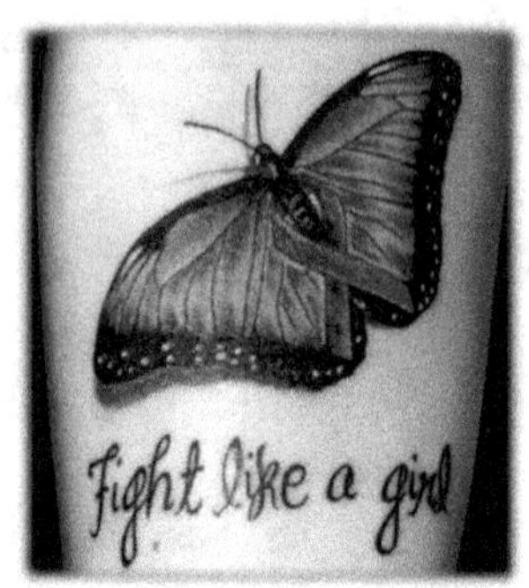

I found a great website, *The Fight Like a Girl Club,* where you can link up with other cancer fighters, survivors and their families. It's a completely free website that allows you to blog and also read the blogs of others. More or less it's a community for anyone who knows anyone battling cancer of any kind.

Finding the website was great, but my first question was "What does it even mean to fight like a girl?" This is what I could find and what I interpreted it to mean.

The country group, Bomshel, proudly chimes out "fight like a girl" in their song of the same name:

"ten years of climbin' that ladder,
all the money and power don't matter
when the doctor said, the cancer spread.
She holds on tight to her husband and her babies,
And says, this is just another test God gave me

And I know how to handle this.
I'll hold my head high
I'll never let this define
The light in my eyes
Love myself, give it hell
Yes, I'll stand and be strong
No, I'll never give up
I will conquer with love
And I'll fight like a girl."

Whether or not someone likes country, the message is transcendent for women everywhere. *Fight like a girl* is a motto, a mantra, that many cancer fighters, survivors, their family and friends have come to be familiar with.

My own personal take on what exactly this statement means? As someone battling Stage III Colon Cancer, it's at the core of who I am. I'm not letting this cancer define me. I'm not going down and I'm damn sure not going down without a fight.

It means no matter how weak or exhausted I am I will *always* give my children the best I have to give. Cancer will not become an excuse for not being able to turn in homework. If I'm legitimately tired from treatment that's one thing. But I absolutely refuse to become someone who constantly says "fill in the blank here...because I have cancer."

Several people, family and strangers alike, believe I shouldn't be traveling to Sicily next month.

They worry because they care, but nothing is keeping me from getting on that plane. People have a tendency to, unintentionally, project their fears onto others in the name of protecting them. To me, *Fight Like a Girl* means never give up, never back down, stay optimistic, be true to yourself - even when the naysayers doubt us. We've got to learn to follow our intuition. It's an exceptionally powerful ally.

Fighting like a girl means you don't let your circumstance define you. You *defy it*, you empower yourself, you use the circumstance as an opportunity for growth and not as a casting call to play the role of victim. It doesn't mean we go completely numb. There are going to be days when we need to cry, need to break things, scream, eat that bowl (or pint) of ice-cream, scribble in our journals until the pen scratches through the pages because we're so angry.

But then we've got to get ourselves back up. Affirm everything that is good in our lives by giving thanks. Even if our health isn't 100% or even 50% of what we want it to be. Hell, if we just sat down and really thought about the grand scheme of things, I think we'd all find that we have more to be thankful for than we have to complain about. Life can still be beautiful in the face of adversity. After all, even when the most severe of storms hit, the sun is still shining when we rise above the clouds.

Saturday - February 8, 2014

My eldest niece took me to get my nose pierced today! She took my hand as I braced myself for the pain. We heard the piercing-gun POP as a diamond stud was forced through my nose.
I've wanted to get it done since I was 15. Felt like such a rebel getting it done today! I know, seems trivial right? Not to me, not now.

The "trivial" moments of life most people overlook are the ones most important to me, especially with what I'm going through. Being there with my niece, experiencing that together, saying YES to doing something I've wanted to do for so long. The small moments are where we define ourselves. Helping a stranger, smiling as we walk past someone in the crowd, appreciating the sunshine. Aren't those moments just as powerful as the bigger ones? They can be when we experience the present moment in a state of gratitude.

This is just the beginning. I want to make this year, my best year. Chemo isn't holding *me* back. I've made a *treatment year bucket list* full of "awesomely fun shit" I'm going to do by the end of the year. Transformational tattoo a few days ago, nose-piercing today, Sicily next month. I've wanted to attend a Dave Matthew's Band concert for as long as I can remember so that's on there too.

Speaking of awesome! My niece surprised me with her new tattoo, in honor of my cancer journey. My name, *Amber,* is written above a colon cancer awareness ribbon with *Strong* below it.

Amber Strong is the nickname they *(my family)* gave me back in December when I was first diagnosed. Her tattoo left me in awe. If that's not a true gesture of unconditional love and emotional support, I don't know what is.

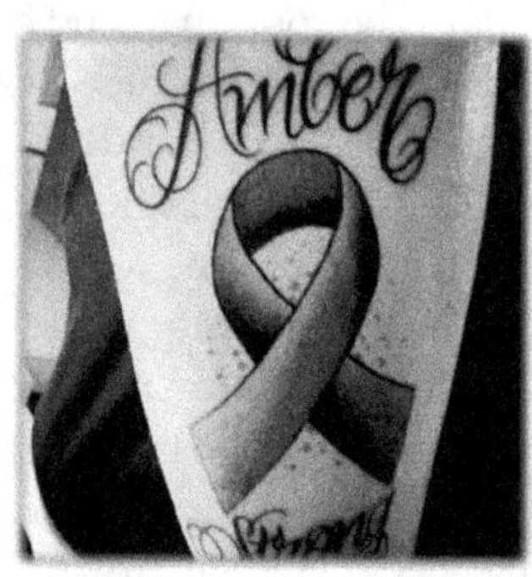

Amber Strong. I like it. Makes me sound like a badass, cancer-fighting, superhero.

I'm learning to laugh at myself more. No, not in a *I'm such a dip shit* way. In a, *I accept myself — nerd humor and all,* way. The first shirt I was going to wear today ended up soaked when Dom took his shower. The second shirt wreaked of oil from being too close to the oil tank on the laundry table for a few days. The third shirt has a broken zipper. By the time I got to the last one, the only thing left to do was laugh.

I thought, *I have to laugh at these discouraging moments. How will I get through chemo if I can't find humor in everyday mishaps?* My burdens are heavy enough without *that* kind of stress.

Sunday - February 9, 2014

Feeling overwhelmed today. Cancer, chemo, no car, financial stress, Felipe, Dom testing boundaries, dipping in and out of depression. It's too much all at once, when everything was looking up. I swear if it wasn't for Dom and Izzy, I wouldn't come back from Italy next month.

My finances are slowly falling to shit. There's money in savings but it will only go so far. No one will hire a cancer patient who can work two weeks per month, when chemo doesn't make me feel like hell.

I've applied for unemployment only to be denied because I was working part time, rather than full time, prior to being diagnosed and didn't accrue enough hours. Disability was also denied because I have a "favorable" prognosis of full remission by the end of the year. SSI benefits seem promising but they're making me jump through countless hoops just to see if I qualify.

Mom was talking to me about applying for public assistance. She said there's nothing wrong with asking for help if you're in need. "It's only temporary, honey, until you get on your feet again."

Welfare? Food stamps? Thinking about it hit me harder than finding out I would need chemotherapy. I've worked so hard *not* to go on it. Depression consumes me most of the time. It's going to kill what's left of my self-confidence to go on public assistance. But my kids *have* to eat, I *have* to eat. The bills can pile up all they want. It's not like my creditors have anything they can take from me. But food, yeah, that's pretty damn important.

Mom has been generous enough to share her vehicle with me but it's been trying. The days I need the car to bring Dom to basketball or martial arts, I have to bring the kids out at 11 p.m. and drop Mom off at work for 2:30 p.m.

I could lose all of my hair from chemo and more weight, even though I'm already underweight at 122 pounds - on a good day. The nurses told me if I drink anything colder than room temperature, it's going to feel like I'm drinking broken glass. Cold temperatures are to be avoided at all costs. I'll have to wear gloves to pour cold juice for the kids and shield my face with a scarf before going in the fridge for anything. Forget about opening the freezer door. Enduring Winter chemo sessions, in New England of all places, is going to take a toll on me if I'm not careful.

Things aren't getting better no matter how grateful I am. Everything is falling to shit. I feel lost, broken, incapable of finding a way to cope. It feels like my life is falling apart at the seams. God, I could use a few less lessons for a while.

The reality of Felipe's absence is settling in. My pain has less to do with him and more to do with

not wanting to go through chemo alone. I'm scared
of not being strong enough for the journey ahead.
Time to let go, process my pain and let the real
healing begin. I've got to, if not for me, for Dom and
Izzy.

Shifting toward gratitude; me and Dom were
able to wake up and watch a whole movie together
before Izzy woke up. In the afternoon, I brought him
to see the new *Frankenstein* movie. About halfway
through *Frankenstein*, we snuck into *The Lego Movie*
instead. Timed it perfectly though! Only missed the
first five minutes.

Dom still wanted more time with me
afterward. Of course I wasn't going to say no. One
day he'll be "too cool" to tell me he loves me in front
of his friends or he'll think it's "weird" to hang out
with me. For now, Dom can be my little shadow all
he wants.

It's hard, some days, knowing I can only do so
much as one parent. I thought about quitting school
to spend more time with them. Only two semesters
left, though, possibly three now. Sicily will be good
for me; mind, spirit and body. I need this trip. I can't
continue on like this, I'm joining a gym. Fuck it.

Monday - February 10, 2014

Today is the first day of bi-weekly meetings with the oncologist. He let me know how my treatments would need to be scheduled for the next six months. Our oncology appointments would be every other Monday, followed by blood work the same day.

Every other Tuesday, the day following my appointment and blood work, will be chemotherapy treatment days.

Tuesday - February 11, 2014
CHEMO SESSION # 1

My port has been accessed, fluids administered and steroids started. Chemo meds will start soon.

The nurse just walked in on me and Mom taking selfies! Kimmy popped in to wish me well and share

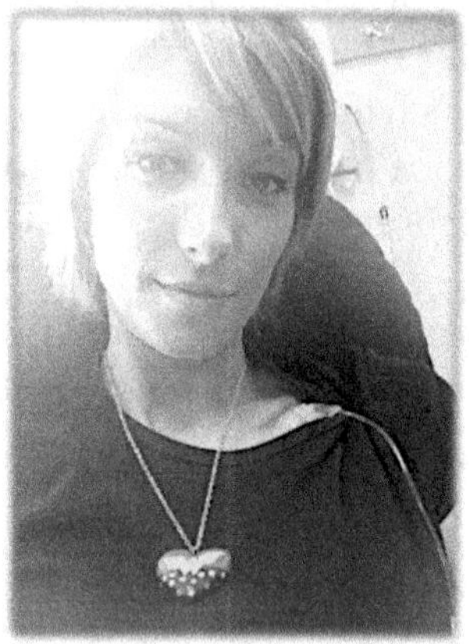

some sister hugs. Thankful for her.

When the nurse accessed my port for the first time it felt like a bee sting, didn't linger for long though. Receiving chemo is pretty damn weird. I have an implant just below my clavicle, there's a needle in it, all kinds of tape wrapped around the outside of it. I feel scared and anxious but other than that, 100 percent healthy. As in, *why am I sitting in this chair, I should go home.* No turning back now.

Think I'll write a poem later, *The Taste of Chemo.* Ugh, the taste was disgusting when the nurse flushed saline through my port. I could taste rubbing alcohol and saline in the back of my throat. She tells me it's *normal.* Something to look forward to. I can hardly contain my excitement for session two. I'm taking a nap.

Later that day...

Chemo is done. Feeling great! Hooked up to a 48-hour chemo pump until Thursday. After four hours of chemo in a chair, I get to wear a fanny-pack lookalike-of-a-purse for the next two days. Good times!

Picking up Iz from daycare, then off to class at UMass tonight! The nurse administered steroids during treatment to help my body absorb the chemo. I'm bouncing off the freaking walls. Thankful for being able to attend class tonight. I'd probably start rearranging furniture in the house if I had to stay home.

Thursday - February 13, 2014

Mom drove us to the hospital today in the middle of a snow storm. Feeling free as a barn swallow now that I'm unhooked from the take-home chemo pump.

She's been phenomenal through it all; putting up with my mood swings, there for major surgery, doctor appointments, helping out with the kids and so much more. She's there to listen when she doesn't agree. No matter how cranky I get, I can cry on her shoulder knowing we'll be just fine. She's my rock.

I'm pretty much in a haze right now. I've been depressed lately. Don't want to go to school anymore, don't want to clean, don't want to cook, don't want to

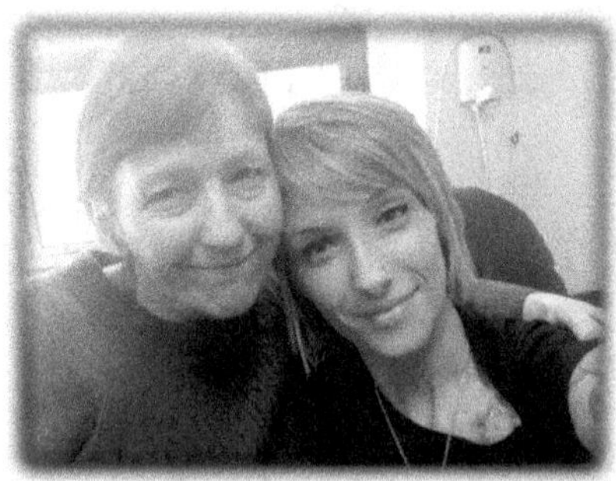

be anywhere anymore. I'm sick of it all.

I love my children so much. I don't want to leave them, not like this. Dominic needs me more than ever right now. What do I do now? How do I get control back over my life?

Handing my well-being over to a group of medical professionals has left me feeling powerless. I'm almost 30 but what have I done with my life? Don't know how to get myself out of this depression. Don't know if I even want to go to school for journalism anymore. I'm lost.

Sunday - February 16, 2014

Feeling pretty hopeless after starting chemo this week until I heard this song by One Republic, *You've Got Something I Need*. It evoked visions of me in a cancer free body where I'm living the life of my dreams. *I'm happy, my body is healthy.*

It gave me hope. Gratitude flooded my mind, filled my heart. What would that look like? What would it *feel* like? To live a purposeful life of intent, helping others, writing, giving, having wild adventures with my kids and seeing them grow into extraordinary adults.

It hit me, we all have this power within us to make a difference. A chance to be the best versions of ourselves. I could feel my own greatness stirring, waking up, *Hey woman! I'm in here, let me out!*

I'm a hot mess, can't tell up from down and don't even know what I'm doing with my life. Still, there must be faith in me on some level. For a moment ever so brief, I was touched by a spark of the divine. I felt peace. I felt surrender.

Monday - February 17, 2014

Fallen back into *that place* again. No motivation, no desire for anything. Assignments are due for class. My room is a mess. Papers are scattered about with haste, clothes here and there. I've wasted so much time…

Saturday - February 22, 2014

Finally feeling like *me* again.

Tuesday - February 25, 2014
CHEMO SESSION # 2

Travel Writing in Sicily purchase receipts came in tonight! Blessed to have received a grant to pay for the trip. I wouldn't be going if it wasn't that grant and financial aid covering the remaining costs. I'm REALLY going to Italy!!!

When I've looked around the room during this session and my last, the other infusion patients appear to be in their fifties, sixties or older. They mostly nap or watch television. There is a tv in 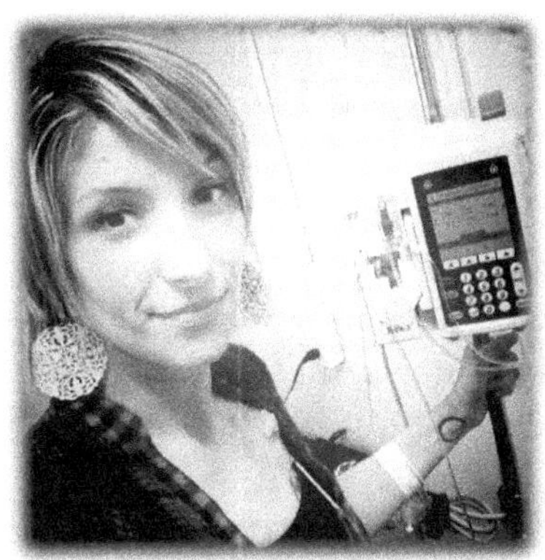 each of our infusion suite areas but I get far too restless to watch anything. Plus, my mom needs a bit of a distraction herself. I'm content with my journal, my laptop and a few books. Although I only lasted an hour last time before falling asleep. Who knows how long I'll last this time.

The patients who are awake, bear forlorn expressions of sadness when they see me sitting in an infusion chair. I'm not accompanying my grandmother for treatment and, although I'm here with my mother, she's thankfully not the patient either. I am.

When the other patients look at me with despair, I smile or wave "hello" or smile *and* wave. I've made it my goal to be *the light* while I'm here, see them smile, have a conversation, share in a laugh or two. I've yet to see anyone younger than me or relatively my age being treated when I'm here.

Heartbreaking, once you understand everyone in here means something to someone, somewhere. Even if they don't currently have family or a person they're close to. At one point and time, they were someone's daughter or son. They may be someone's sibling, aunt, uncle, mother or father. My story is one of many. Each of us in this room has a story to tell. Patients, nurses, doctors; we all do.

The Universe gives us all these experiences to grow from and opportunities for connection. I won't miss going through chemo when all is said and done. I will miss chatting with nurses, being here with fellow cancer patients. They're absolute angels. Each treatment leaves me feeling more connected to them, more supported on this journey and more loved.

4
MARCH 2014
Famiglia

> *"Family is not an important thing,*
> *it's everything."*
> ~Michael J. Fox

Sunday - March 2, 2014

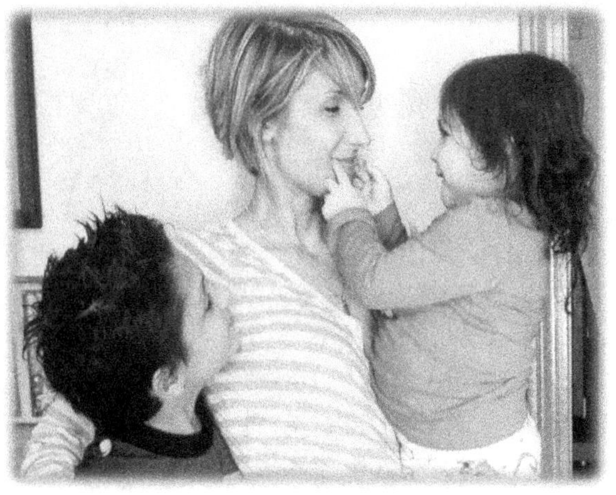

Looked over at Izzy today and told her, "You're my little princess." She responded with, "No I'm not mommy. I'm queen of the castle." She's already so much confident than I was as a child. Full of wisdom. Thankful for her dynamic, strong-willed personality. She has as much to teach *to* me, as she has to learn *from* me.

Friday - March 7, 2014

One week from today I'll be in sunny Sicily! At least, I think it's sunny there? Even if it rains every day, I love rainstorms. This is really happening! Scheduled to have chemo this coming Tuesday but Mom recommends me waiting until I get back and she's right. I shouldn't be flying out of the country days after receiving treatment.

Dom and Izzy had me laughing so hard, today, my belly hurt. Dom was pretending to sleep in my bed so Izzy wouldn't bother him. That idea fell short when Izzy developed a plan of her own to wake him up. "Hey Mommy, I got an idea! We can play drums to wake up Domigick!"

She marched on over to the cabinet, pulled out two metal cook pot lids and ran up to her "sleeping" brother and clanged them together inches away from his face. He was a great sport though, kept laughing and laughing. Thank you, God, for these moments.

Thursday - March 13, 2014

Somehow found the energy to bring Dom and Izzy to the local children's museum. The insurmountable joy I felt watching them chase after one another, laughing, playing, being kids was priceless. For a few short hours I didn't feel like a cancer patient. I felt like a Mom. Sacred.

Within the walls of that museum, we shared sacred space. My cancer diagnosis wasn't allowed to enter, nor was fatigue or chemo or my depression. Only love, laughter and the memories of time well spent with family. Thank you for today.

Saturday - March 15, 2014

First impressions of Mama Sicilia

… the mountain, a sleeping giant that greets you as you step off the plane in Palermo.

Earthen clad spikes of rock protrude up through the ground…

…undulating green mountains, their base adorned by terra cotta stucco houses…

This place, so vastly different from home. Turquoise waters, drink in warm air, let it wash

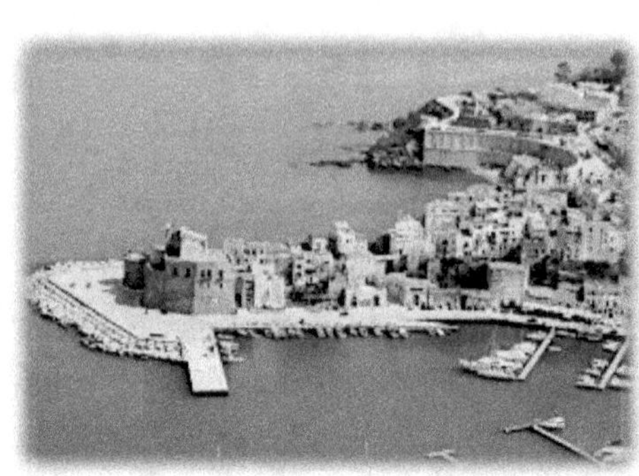

over you, nourishing your soul. Gone are the frigid temperatures of home. Birds chirping, cars pass above us on the main road. A motor bike zooms by with the rhythmic humming buzz of a giant, mechanical bee.

Water mimics sky, though the sea is bluer and deeper. Several sailboats, below us, adorn the docks of the bay.

"Arancini," sticky, polenta-like, rice balls made of corn, stuffed with tomatoes and onion. Hand-made miniature pistachio cannoli's.

temple ruins of Selinunte

...thousands of years after Greeks built the temple, here it stands. Columns scattered in the distance as though Zeus himself dismantled Hera's temple. Fluted stone sections cast out one by one, in a fit of heated rage to spite the *Queen of the Gods.*

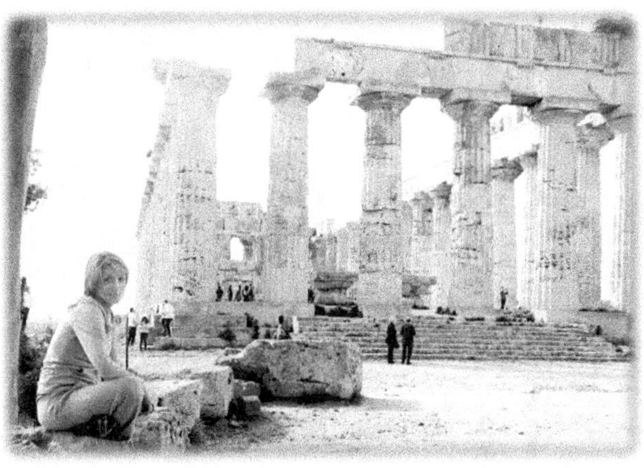

Tuesday - March 18, 2014

The people of Castelbuono have received us with a wonderfully warm welcome. They appreciate when we speak their native tongue, even if our Italian is slightly broken up by words in English we lack the Italian counterpart for. Their eyes light up with amazement and joy, pure pride, when we take interest in what they're selling. They openly share their lives with us and in return we carry a piece of their culture, their history and their stories back with us to America.

Thursday - March 20, 2014

This week has been a treasure trove of wonder; rich food, captivating culture and the people of Sicily who make us feel like *famiglia*. Traveling from one side of this island *paradiso* to the other has been magic.

I've climbed the craters of an active volcano, skinny-dipped in the Mediterranean, woke at dawn for sunrise yoga on the beach. Let's not forget Vitamin D therapy on the brown-sugar-texture beach of Cefalù,

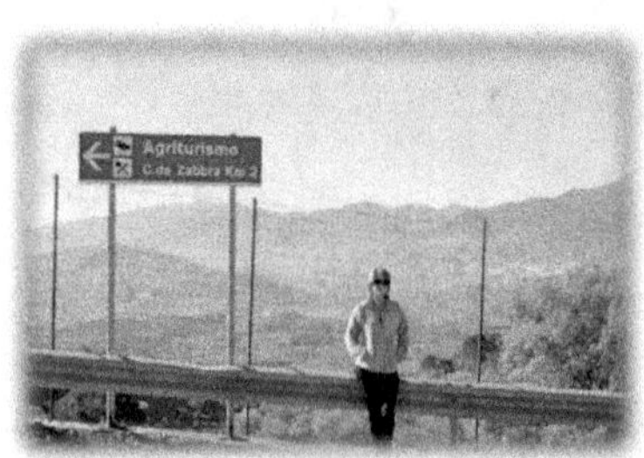

discussing ancient history with a handsome Sicilian *(we'll call "Marco')*. My spirit was sanctified by the rich beauty of this island, long before that rather handsome Sicilian took me out tonight, just the two of us.

Marco drove us around Siracusa, bestowing tales of its history with that beguiling accent of his. He spoke of history being "written by the winners," the conquerors. Our conversation transitioned to the topic of travel. He told me, "If we were meant to stay in one place, we would have been given roots."

We parked the car along the boardwalk, continuing our chat as we walked together, stopping at a few restaurants. It wasn't enough to simply "eat pizza together" as most American men would have done back home. Marco spoke passionately of his culture; explaining why tomatoes, fresh mozzarella and basil were used *and why* when creating the very first *Margherita* pizza.

Our conversation over wine and "pie" felt like a scene taken from the movie *Under the Tuscan Sun* with Diane Lane. I opened up to him about my concern with raising a boy on my own, as a woman. He paused for a moment, picked a fork up from the table and stood it upright so the prongs reached toward the sky. "You see this fork? This is like a tree. If you plant a stick here with the tree, the tree grows straight. But if you wait to put the stick in later, once the tree has already begun to bend, it's too late."

Marco provided parenting advice with poetic eloquence. His accent kept me spellbound, my adoration transcending the superficial. Something in the way he moved, the way he carried himself, it was mesmerizing. Proud yet humble, educated but not arrogant. Seductive *and* respectful. Marco is the cliché embodiment of men abroad who American women swoon over. I love Sicily.

Friday - March 21, 2014

I climbed Mt. Etna today! Think I'll add that one to my *treatment year bucket list*! Hundreds, perhaps thousands, of ladybugs crawled at my feet and flew around - feeding on minerals in the volcanic rock. Etna is

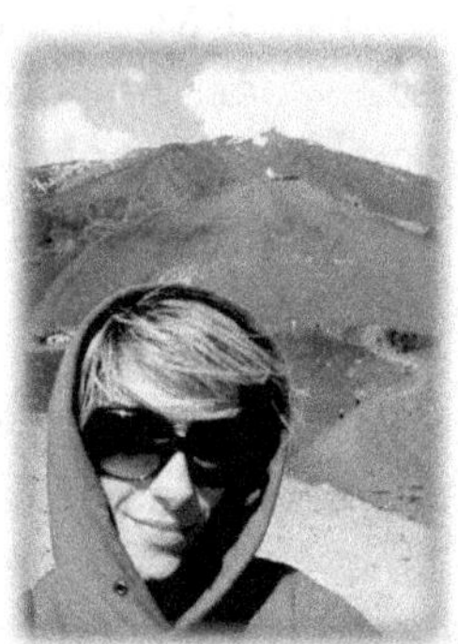

referred to in the feminine, as equally as she is revered by native Sicilians. Our class broke off in groups so we could explore several of her craters on our own.

The coolest moment for me was when I called Dom and Izzy, "Guess where Mommy is? I'm at the top of Mt. Etna! It's a volcano here in Sicily!" They asked if I could bring home a few pieces of volcanic rock. Our tour guide told us that, unlike in Hawaii, Sicilians actually *want* tourists to bring pieces of rock home because they have it in excess. Sicilians ship it out to be used in crop soil. It paves their roads. They use it to make bracelets and other souvenirs all over their Mediterranean island.

Heading to the *Time Out Pub* in Taormina with my classmates tonight once we're all ready to go. They're going to help me "de-mom" my wardrobe and I'm all for it!

I didn't know what to expect coming into this class, being nearly ten years a senior to my classmates. Never once have they made me feel like the "mom" of the group. Never once have they excluded me or treated me differently because of the age difference. If anything, they've made me feel like one of the "kids." I have to laugh because there's been a few times when they've come out and said "I keep forgetting you're a mom!" Meaning I don't fit their stereotypical mom description, but in a good way.

What an amazing group of students, every one of them. I'm honored to share this adventure with them.

Saturday - March 22, 2014

Last night I stayed up until nearly 4 a.m. with two of my classmates. After we left *La Giara Nightclub*, there was a drunken escapade involving a shoulder ride up to an orange tree, where we attempted to pick fruit that was (unbeknownst to us) prolifically sour.

We climbed to the rooftop of our hotel after, drinking Planeta red wine, gazing off in admiration at Etna. Our professors said it's been years since She erupted during one of these annual class trips. Yet, there we were, mesmerized by a steady flow of red-orange lava pulsing forth from Etna's mouth. Amazing.

Monday - March 24, 2014

Dieci giorni in paradiso, more memories than can be counted.
Now it's back to reality. Bloodwork today, chemo tomorrow. Happy to see at my weigh-in this morning I've gained nearly six pounds while in Italy! Wish it were ten pounds since chemo takes such a toll on me.

Grateful for a magnificent journey in Sicilia, for the amazing people I bonded with along the way. I'll think of Sicily when my treatment, and life in general, gets to be too much.

Have decided to go pixie with my hair and return to being a brunette. My hair has been falling out like crazy. Brings me to tears when I see clumps of it in the shower. Better to go shorter now, in case chemo leaves me bald, than be even more traumatized later.

When I started cutting my hair shorter in December, I did it because I thought I might have cancer. Never told anyone that. I was afraid my hair would fall out if I needed chemo. That's the real reason I cut off ten inches. Since it's *actually* falling out now, what's four or five more?

Before traveling to Sicily, I needed to write a feature story of my choosing about local food. One of our local farms is nationally-known for its famous apple cider donuts. After emailing the president of the farm, a few of my classmates and me stopped in to be part of their donut making process.

The president of the farm must have been impressed because she emailed me this morning, asking to publish it on the front page of their monthly newsletter! WOOT WOOT!

Tuesday - March 25, 2014
CHEMO SESSION # 3
weight: 126.6 pounds/57.42 kilograms
{Dominic's Birthday}

Five years ago, today, a fighter was born. He stormed into this big scary new world five weeks and two days early, ready to take action. He's given me strength when I've had none, taught me to have patience when I didn't know I had it in me.

God knows it hasn't been easy lately. The last three months or so have been incredibly trying. But I will take every time he talks back, yells at me or refuses to do his chores over not having him here to do any of those things or not being here to witness them. When I count my blessings, Dominic is at the very top of that list.

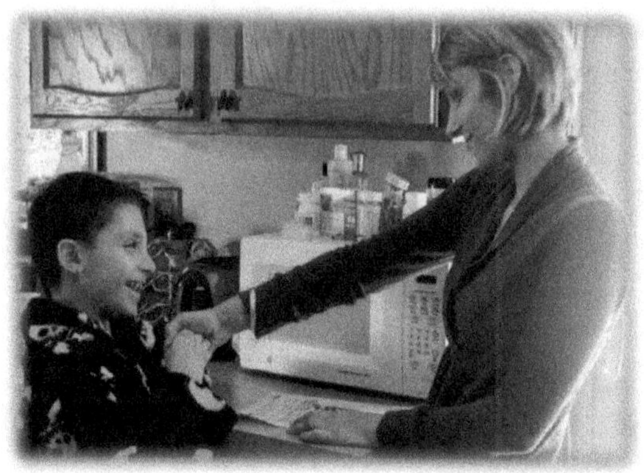

Other blessings include the company I've had thus far to make the time pass during treatments. My mom was with me for treatments one and two. She wasn't missing them for anything.

My sister, Kim, coincidentally has a friend going through the same situation as me. Her friend had surgery a few weeks after I had mine. We both started chemotherapy on the same day for the same type of cancer. Our treatments coincide which means Kim usually visits with both of us. Seeing my sister's smile is like warm sunshine. I don't give a shit if it does sound cheesy to say it, I love having her here with me.

My last treatment, a close personal friend of mine came up to the third floor infusion suite to visit. His personality overflows with good vibes, always finding just the right words when a friend or family is in need. Having been through a traumatic ordeal of his own a few years back, any advice he has to offer comes from experience. I'm always eager to listen.

Kay, one of the nurses, always offers me Ativan as part of the treatment. I usually decline because of the night class at UMass but I don't have any homework tonight and my nerves are jumpy. I just got back from Sicily two days ago. I'm really not looking forward to another treatment. So for today, I'm taking the damn Ativan.   Hopefully a good nap will get me through this.

Wednesday - March 26, 2014

This morning, after ten days of enjoying gelato to die for, I completely forgot about having extreme sensitivity to cold after chemo. Without thinking, I went into the fridge to grab a gallon of chocolate milk. My fingers didn't start tingling right away when I grabbed the handle to remind me I'm a chemo patient. I poured a glass and down the hatch it went.

It was like chugging an ice cold glass of milk after eating an entire bag of peppermints mixed with shards of broken glass. Chemo cold rush makes a brain freeze feel like a soothing cranial massage. The pain is *that* bad. My throat felt like it was closing up on me. Damn near dropped the glass of milk when I ran to the faucet for hot water. Once I chugged the hot water down, my pain subsided. The pins and needles went away. It's just *great* to be home.

Thursday - March 27, 2014

In serious need of decompression. Chemo left me wiped out this week. My Mom is my hero. She noticed how exhausted I am, went into work late, picked Izzy up from daycare and met Dom at the bus stop after school. All so I can sleep. As stubborn as I can be, today, I am so accepting help.

5
APRIL 2014
Reality

> *"We do not run when the volcano erupts.*
> *Actually, we run toward it."*
> *~una donna di Sicilia*

Tuesday - April 1, 2014

Created a *Go Fund Me* page to start saving up for a vehicle of my own. What a struggle it was to make that decision! Asking for help (and receiving it) has been tremendously difficult for me. Especially in matters of finance. I feel like this is my life, and if I've gotten myself into a financial conundrum, *I* should be the one to pull my ass out of it.

At a certain point, though, you realize you're actually in quicksand. The more wiggling you do to get out of it, the faster you're pulled in. Time to extend a lifeline and ask for help.

Wednesday - April 2, 2014

My friend Angela surprised me with a little care package in the mail today! Handmade bows for

Izzy, a mini-top-hat and two barrettes for me. One of the barrettes bears a pin that says "fight like a girl." Brightened my day when the package came in from her. Who doesn't love receiving gifts in the mail?

Took the kids out to the park, and the dog, who climbed up the play scape and went down the slide. Family, nature, laughter. They have become my biggest healers.

Saturday - April 5, 2014

Found Aranciatta Rosso at the grocery store tonight! Going to close my eyes and go back to Sicily as I savor every sip. Little things like this keep me going.

Dom was watching tv today when he said "Mom! You got to see this commercial, the mom dances just like you!" Vanilla Ice, the musician, was with a random mom in the grocery store aisle who (clearly) was dancing like no one else is watching. Her son stands there, staring at her in total embarrassment.

Neither one of us could hold back our laughter. The little boy in the commercial reacted the same way Dom would have in that situation and the mom was 100 percent me.

Go ninja, go ninja go!

Tuesday - April 8, 2014
CHEMO SESSION # 4

It's Tuesday morning. Chemo time. *Kay*, my nurse, hasn't begun the chemo portion of my treatment yet. She's accessed my port, which means a butterfly needle has been inserted through skin into my Porta Cath. A bag of dextrose hangs from the intravenous pole next to me.

Haven't been given steroids, anti-nausea meds, chemo or the 5FU flush yet. I believe they named it the 5FU flush because it's given last after all of the other medications. Maybe they thought it would be a funny play on words since chemo makes patients feel that way after treatment, "F U."

I look to Mom, contently reading *Dear Abby*. "Hey Mom," I ask her, "do they spell dear Abby with a y or with an i?" She replies "y", so I say "*Why?* Because I asked you." We both laugh. She smiles at me with that "love you sweetheart, I'm going to laugh so I don't cry" look in

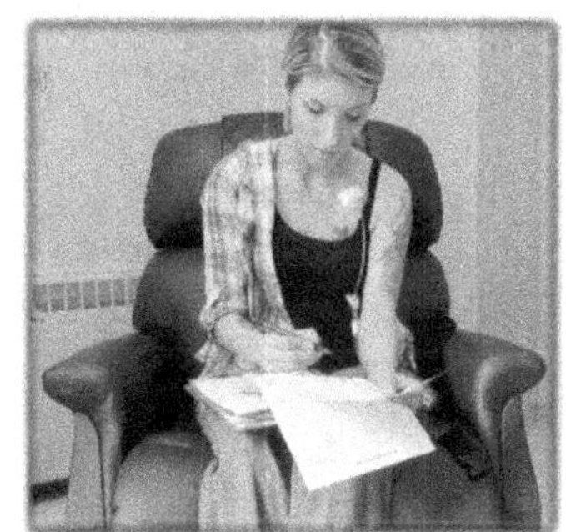

her eyes. The look of a mother accompanying her daughter to chemotherapy.

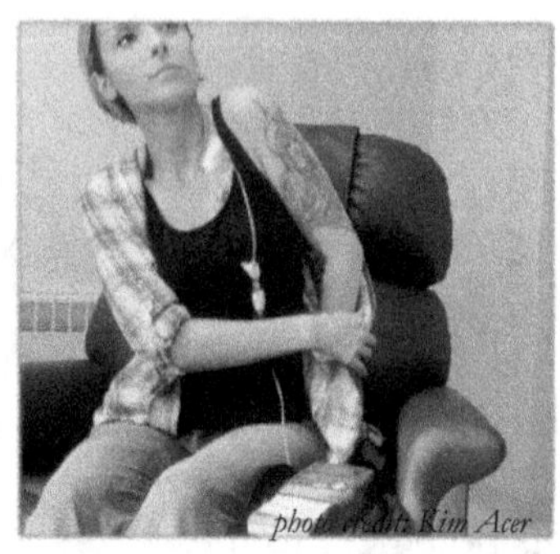

Treatment is about to begin, but I'll maintain my nerdy sense of humor if it means Mom thinks I'm doing okay, if it means *she'll* be okay.

Didn't want to come in today for treatment. I'm tired of it already. I feel healthy, I feel strong. I don't feel like a cancer patient. My blood counts have been perfect, *knock on wood,* when they've been checked the day before treatment.

I've seen blogs and read stories, like *Chris Beat Cancer,* about people who miraculously cure themselves without ever needing chemo or surgery. Our mind is an exceptionally powerful tool with unlimited potential if we learn how to tap into it. Unfortunately, I haven't gotten to that place in my journey…yet.

I've decided to pair the non-traditional approach of Reiki, exercise and juicing with the traditional treatment of chemo, surgery and *trying* to reduce stress to a minimum. I wish I had been given more time to make my decision. Everything happened so fast when I was diagnosed. Part of me wishes I had only undergone surgery. That I had turned to holistic medicine and extreme dietary changes, rather than chemo.

Doctors felt my cancer was moving aggressively. Too aggressively to wait. I didn't have time to think about alternative therapies let alone research them with the way they moved the course of my treatment along. I don't know that I *would* have made it without surgery. The tumor in my colon wasn't just bleeding, it was hemorrhaging.

After surgery, the tumor that was removed from my colon was sent out for genetic testing. There was no genetic link whatsoever between my family and colon cancer. None.

There's a reason why colon cancer diagnoses for people my age, in their late twenties, is on the rise. There's so much shit in the food we eat; chemical preservatives, dyes, chemicals we shouldn't be putting into our body. Don't even get me started on genetically modified foods (GMO's).

Sitting in a chemo chair for hours on end has given me ample time to research chemicals found in products all over the U.S. - from the food and drink we consume to the products we're using in our homes. Parabens, polyparabens and sulfates in our hygiene products, makeup, self-tanning lotions, lotion in general. Tetra sodium EDTA, Butylated Hydroxytoluene (BHT), Aluminum in our deodorant.

ABC News published an online article, *11 Food Ingredients Banned Outside the U.S. that We Eat,* listing 11 such ingredients banned in other countries and what scientists have to say about them. Ingredients like Blue #1, banned in Norway and France, brominated vegetable oil found in soda and sports drinks and others.

One can literally get lost down the rabbit hole of information, there's so much to look into and read. In the end, what it comes down to is our responsibility as consumers. There seems to be no shortage of food processed with chemicals in our country. Yet there are healthy options too. Is it more expensive? Yes. Of course it is. Aren't our bodies worth it though?

My grandfather used to have this saying, "You get what you pay for." We pay next to nothing for the price of food, then we're going to get shit food that can potentially harm our bodies. It's a bit different in the world of health and beauty where even the pricy cosmetics can contain chemicals banned in other countries for having carcinogenic properties.

Refinery29.com posted an article stating there are currently 1, 372 chemicals banned from cosmetics in the Europe but only ten banned in the U.S. Ten. Are you fucking kidding me? *(present day note: Cancer.gov also contains articles expressing the highly possible connection between aluminum based antiperspirants and breast cancer)*

Before knowing about all these chemicals, I started making the transition in our household a few years back to organic, non-GMO living. Dom drives my mom crazy, sometimes, checking the ingredient labels of food she keeps in the house. "Grandma! Do you know what's in this stuff? High fructose corn syrup? Hydrog-gen-ga-nated oils? Mali-something, I can't even pronounce this! Grandma, this is so bad for you, it's like poison in a box!" She'll look at me with slight disdain, saying, "Here we go again."

I'm almost at the end of my treatment for today. I've been given Decadron, a steroid that aids in the absorption of chemo. Emend, an anti-nausea medication. Oxaliplatin, one of the chemo meds, which can only be given through the dextrose flush line. Leucovorin will be next, then the 5FU flush at the end. But now, it's time for lunch. Mom's homemade shepherd's pie. She even used organic ingredients because she knew I wouldn't eat it otherwise. Nothing like comfort food from home on chemo days.

Wednesday - April 9, 2014

There is so much potential to be unlocked within the human mind. Optimism is one of the most important weapons cancer patients can have.

The first response people typically give me when they hear I've been diagnosed with cancer is "I'm so sorry to hear that" or "That's terrible." There's also the "negative, thank you for making me feel like a walking corpse statements." To which my reply is, "Thank you, I appreciate your concern but this is just another thing for me to overcome."

Everyone deals with these kinds of things in their own way. It's a natural human response when we hear something *we perceive* as devastating to say we're sorry for someone. It's just our way of showing empathy for what they're going through. Honestly, telling someone we love "I'm so sorry" isn't a terrible response.

There's been a lot of wonderful advice from friends and family. There's also been unwarranted concerns about certain things; my traveling out of the country, going to the gym, working on my degree. When people start to tell me I'm pushing myself or in denial of my circumstance, based on a projection of their own fears - that's where I rather diplomatically draw the line. If they're not in this body, thinking with this brain, they shouldn't presume to know what's best for me. I'm the only one that can make that judgement call.

Thursday - April 10, 2014

Raised $1,020.00 on Go Fund Me toward a vehicle. YES! Feeling wiped out but pulling it together for my kiddos. Izzy has an art show tonight at preschool and Dom has open house. Thankful for these babes giving me something to look forward to. Something to focus on outside myself.

Friday - April 11, 2014

In less than two weeks a little over $1,000 has been raised toward the cost of getting me and the kids into a dependable vehicle! It's going to help us in so many ways; transportation, stress relief from scheduling conflicts, stress relief for parents. They've stepped up in so many ways, accommodating the needs of me and Dom and Izzy. This means more independence for me, more time to focus on healing my physical body.

None of this would have been possible without friends and family donating to my cause. Couldn't do this without everyone, feel abundantly blessed to be surrounded by so many caring people.

Saturday - April 12, 2014

Bowling tonight with Izzy, Dom, Kim, Lisa and all of our munchkins! Sister time is one of my absolute favorite times. Can't wait!

Sunday - April 13, 2014

Attended a Goo Goo Dolls concert at UMass tonight with some classmates. Phenomenal! To think this Fall I'll be a senior.

Wednesday - April 16, 2014

Krista, my friend from Virginia, thought I went to bed while she was driving all night to visit me. Nope! Too excited to see her. Glad she's here, feeling pretty loved and lucky to have her in my life.

Thursday - April 17, 2014

Today was my last visit with Dr. Roes. I'm done. Not with treatment but with being treated like every other patient he has. I'm not an 80-year-old woman or a 60-year-old man. I don't want to be prescribed another medication every damn time I start experiencing a new side effect. *You've got anxiety and insomnia from the steroids, here's a prescription for Ativan.* Replaced that with meditation, Reiki and gratitude. *You're experiencing neuropathy and pins and needles, here's a prescription for pain.* Replaced that with holistic herbal remedies. *You're experiencing nausea, here's a script for Zofran.* Replaced that with holistic herbal remedies as well.

Today was the last straw. I've been severely constipated because of chemo. Suppose I'm fortunate. From what the nurses tell me, most patients experience extreme bouts of diarrhea from the same treatment. I checked in with Dr. Roes today and let him know. *Here's a prescription for Miralax*, he says. Miralax? As in the laxative that contains Polyethylene glycol? Yeah, no. That's not going to work for me buddy.

I ask Dr. Roes about Senna tea. I've read online it's supposed to be helpful for constipation. He looks at me and tells me my gut can become dependent on Senna and that "This is what we always prescribe for patients with constipation. It's what we've always prescribed because it works." I expressed that I live as holistically as possible. My family eats organically grown, local, farm fresh food. The products we use at home are chemical and dye free.

I asked if he could recommend any herbal or all natural remedies. He said, "You're all natural? But you're going through chemo aren't you? Not very natural now is it? Use the Miralax, it's what's recommended." My blood was boiling. The hairs on the back of my neck stood up. It took every bit of personal restraint not to leap out of my chair and pull a Homer Simpson on him. He would be Bart in that reference.

Dr. Roes walked out of the office and I headed straight for the front desk. My two favorite girls were working. "I need a new oncologist." They both looked at me, wide-eyed, wondering what had transpired during my office visit. One of them asked who my oncologist was. When I informed her and explained what happened, she looked at me reassuringly. "You're not the first patient to voice those concerns."

I took a deep breath of gratitude in and exhaled a long, slow sigh of relief. It brought me comfort to know I wasn't alone. She recommended Dr. Scho. He's family oriented and much warmer than Dr. Roes. I hope she's right.

Monday - April 21, 2014

Brought Dom to see *Captain America: Winter Soldier* today! Love having this time with my boy. Growing up on Marvel Comics, I never imagined having such a cool kid to watch the movies with. Although I can't say I imagined the comics would become an epic movie series either.

I'd like to start doing more for myself, to nourish my spirit and stay focused during chemo. Just so I don't forget, I've created a list.

Here goes:

• Continue going to healing events; group meditations, Reiki sessions, energy healing programs, etc. They nurture my soul, mind and physical body. They encourage me to continue growing and evolving on a deep soul level.

• Stop being so hard on myself. Yes, I'm 29 and live with my mom but I'm working toward owning a vehicle, finishing my degree, raising two children and kicking cancer's ass! Who gives a shit what other people think or say - this is *my* life. I have to live it to the fullest. For myself, for Dom, for Izzy. Take time to see the significance of your life, how magnificent you are, how magnificent we all are. There is greatness within you, let it shine.

• Let love in. Wild, passionate, powerful love. Love that transcends what our minds are capable of understanding. Not romantic love with a partner, rather, unconditional love for the woman you are becoming. Embrace her, forgive her, honor her, love her and in the process - fall effortlessly in love with a life you're thankful to be living.

• Keep moving forward, embrace change and make peace with where you are in life. You are *exactly* where you are meant to be.

Wednesday - April 23, 2014

No chemo this week, platelets are too low. The day before treatment my oncologist runs a panel of blood work to see if my body is strong enough to handle the next day's chemotherapy treatment. The panel, called a CBC or complete blood count, measures the number of white cells, platelets, red blood cells and hemoglobin present. Sometimes my oncologist will check my magnesium levels as well just in case.

My platelet count is in the high sixties this week which means chemo is a no go for this week. Normal range for a healthy person is about 130. The lowest an oncologist will accept is 75. Anything below that can cause internal bleeding if chemo is administered. This is the first time health concerns have delayed treatment. Hoping they'll be back up next week. Want to get through this as soon as I can.

I keep seeing Robins everywhere; on the deck, in the driveway, at my window, on the fence post. They speak to me of creativity and new beginnings. Connecting with nature is one of the little comforts that brings me peace.

Sunday - April 27, 2014

Traveled to Brooklyn to visit the *Brooklyn Botanical Garden* with Dom, Mom and a few of Mom's friends from work. I'm exhausted but the trip was entirely worth it. It's no coincidence combining the words "great" and "attitude" pretty much create the word "gratitude."

Thankful for today. The air we breathe is a blessing.

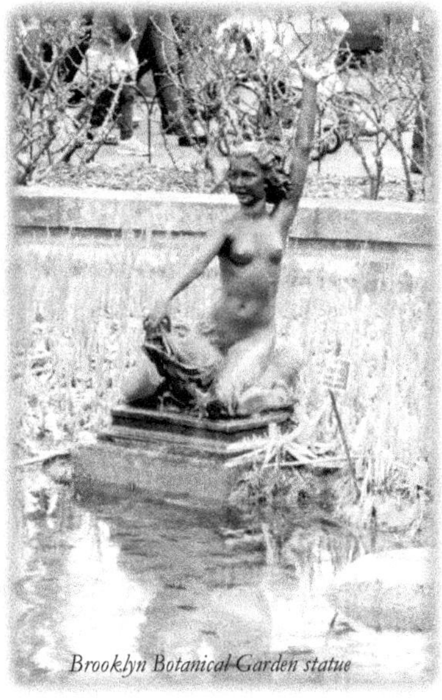

Brooklyn Botanical Garden statue

Tuesday - April 29, 2014
CHEMO SESSION # 5

Each of us face personal battles throughout our lifetimes. That journey is different for everyone. For some it can be job loss, a loved one passing away, disease, raising children alone, coming out to the world, staying true to themselves. For others it's not so much a battle as it can be a learning experience.

The idea is not to say "my struggle is greater than yours" or "he/she has it so much better than me." The point is to grow through it, to inspire others with our strength, with our challenges, to forgive ourselves and others, heal, awaken our soul. Find our own strengths by tapping into the better, brighter parts of ourselves that we didn't know were there. We *all* have it within us.

Chemo session five was rough today. The physical side effects were relatively minor—some nausea and fatigue, typical treatment side effects. The steroids paired with treatment, however, threw me for a loop. I only receive steroids the day of treatment but they can stay in my system for days. Which means out of the blue, my heart will start racing as though someone just gave me a dose of adrenaline. Steroids create an insatiable appetite, bring on jitters and cause my heart to race. All before making me feel like I want to clean the entire house top to bottom and rearrange furniture.

During treatment I watched the movie by Louise Hay, *You Can Heal Your Life*. It focuses on why controlling your thoughts, as well as the emotion and energy behind them, is so important. Functioning on "autopilot" as I call it, is what most of us do on a day to day basis. We get so caught up in the mundane, living life on repetition. Stuck in that place it's easy to wonder, *will it ever change? When is my life going to begin?*

Living an awakened life doesn't mean we have to sit for weeks under the Bodhi tree to attain enlightenment, as Siddhartha did becoming Buddha. It just means waking the heck up. Living in the moment. Realizing we are so much more than this *shell* of a human being. I truly believe, with conviction, we are spiritual beings having a human experience on this earth. It's okay to experience shit days as long as we don't choose to *live* there.

Speaking of shit days...

After chemo I was irritable, moody, exhausted and wired at the same time. My mood is only worsening as the day progresses. Hormones from my monthly cycle are adding an avalanche of emotional mood swings to my already fatigued body. I want to cry for no reason. I've gotten angry and irritated with something as trivial as misplacing something I needed. I enjoy my own company; have since I was a child. Not today though. I'd like to crawl out of my skin and leave the *other* Amber far behind.

I'm fortunate to be surrounded by such a strong support system. I've never been closer to my parents, my siblings and some of my friends as I am now.

Dom and Izzy have kept me firmly rooted, as a sea of chaos rages within me. They give me reasons to get out of bed in the morning, beyond needing me to get them ready for the day.

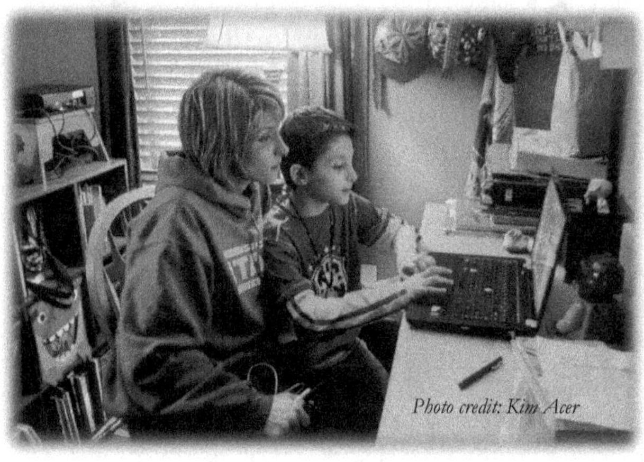

Photo credit: Kim Acer

No greater joy than when my little humans run to greet me at the door, squeezing breath from my chest and the bones in my body beneath bear hugs. Their love lends me strength to keep fighting.

Wednesday - April 30, 2014

Dom is (willingly) having a tea party in the living room with Izzy. I should check for a fever or make sure aliens haven't replaced him with a pod person. Izzy is teaching me yoga. Tea parties and yoga in my living room. Life is good.

6
MAY 2014
Keep Moving Forward

> *"Your thoughts become your words,*
> *your words become your actions*
> *and your actions become your destiny."*
> *~Ghandi*

Thursday - May 1, 2014

Ugh, steroids have had me moody and irritable the last few days! Getting my pump detached today, thank God. Thankful my parents have been as patient as they have been this week. I don't even like being around me when I feel like this.

Friday - May 2, 2014

Today is a new day, seize the moment. Find gratitude in the smallest of moments. For they are what matter most.

...the huge smile on Izzy's face when I pick her up from daycare, the way she runs over to me with open arms, Dom's excitement and extreme goofiness after a great baseball

practice, tucking them in at night, waking up to snuggles in the morning, butterfly eyelash kisses...

Wednesday - May 7, 2014

The mother-daughter relationship I share with Mom has begun to heal since my diagnosis. It's drawn us closer together but there are still so many things left unsaid. Wounds that have yet to be healed, on both our parts. The mother-child relationship is powerful, both as a healer and a teacher. It impacts our lives in ways we can only begin to imagine. Many triggers are present, but many moments for connection and growth as well.

Saturday - May 10, 2014

Trying to type up and piece together a large portfolio of writing for class. Dom and Izzy are both home and have picked today of all days to continuously antagonize one another. Izzy has been intermittently clinging to my back like a baby Koala.

Attempting to get any real work done with them in the house is the equivalent of brushing my teeth while eating cookies. Sure it seems like a good idea at first but the practicality of it is lacking entirely.

Sunday - May 11, 2014

Had an extra-long stay in the massage chair at the gym this morning. Spent the day at the beach with Mom, Dom and Izzy. Stopped on the way home for dinner at a Greek Pizzeria. Grabbed ice cream to go and headed home. Babes are sleeping, with this tired mama soon to follow. Can't get much better than spending it seaside with the ones I love. Happy Mother's Mom. Love you.

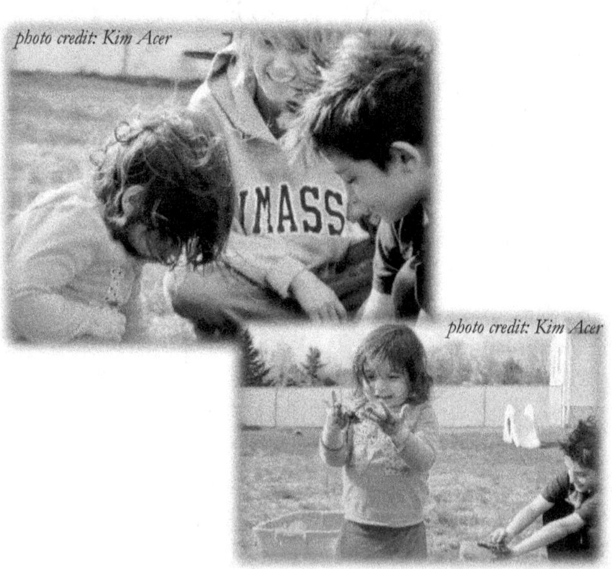

Monday - May 12, 2014

First oncology check-in with Dr. Scho today. He walked in the room with a smile, greeted me with a solid handshake and began asking the ages of my children right away. He asked what I was going to school for, how my classes were going and said one of his children had gone to school for journalism ages ago. He pulled up pictures of his grandchildren on his phone. I did the same with photos of Dom and Izzy. The receptionist was right. I'm going to be much happier with Dr. Scho as my oncologist moving forward.

I've been quite pleased with how well my gym workouts have been coming along too. I never, and I mean *never*, thought I would join a gym. Right after the divorce I was dating someone for a few months who was a total "gym rat." Once he got out of work, he'd work out for an hour or so before coming over to spend time with me. Once or twice he asked if I would ever go to the gym with him. I remember having a bit of laugh about it, thinking, *Is he out of his damn mind? I'm not joining a gym. He must be crazy.*

At that time, I didn't know anything about fitness or how certain training programs enhance or shape a person's physique. *If I only weigh 120 pounds now,* I thought, *what's going to happen if I join the gym? My body looks fine just the way it is.* Had I known of the countless benefits; from how you feel mentally to what it does to your energy levels, to the anti-aging properties on a cellular level, to the boost in self-confidence it delivers when you start to see results - I would have run to the closest gym.

A major component of personal resistance was my lack in self-confidence as. I was completely intimidated by the idea of joining a gym. The thought of walking into a gym, where there were tons of guys working out and me not knowing what the hell I'm supposed to do or how - practically brought on a panic attack just to think about it.

The only thing that mattered after that cancer diagnosis was returning my body to a state of optimal health. Living long enough and becoming strong enough to be there for my babes. I didn't give a shit about anyone watching me workout or what they might think. Cancer made my irrational fears and insecurities feel insignificant in comparison.

Joining the gym two months ago has changed my life. It's given me heightened energy levels, more confidence and expanded my self-love. I'm able to walk with my shoulders back, head held high because I feel healthier, happier, stronger. Thank you, cancer, for trying to take my life. All you're doing is making me stronger.

Tuesday - May 13, 2014

Chemo session six canceled for today. Delayed until next week, as long as labs are better. Platelets too low, once again. All of my other blood cell counts are

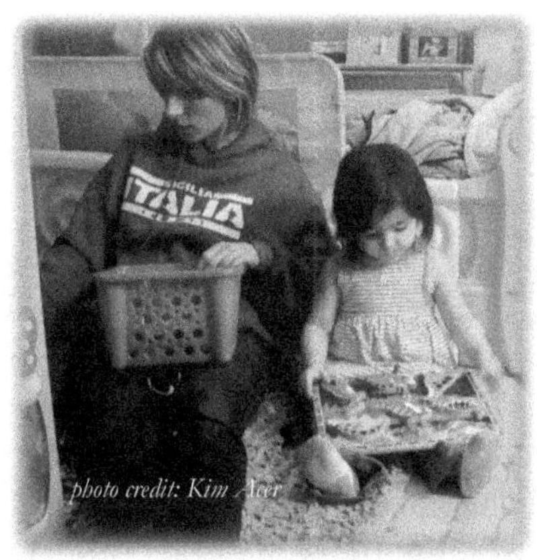

photo credit: Kim Acer

right where they should be. Good thing chemo was canceled. Little Miss Iz is running a fever with a terrible cough. Bringing my peanut to the doctor's today.

Best entertainment for a high energy two-year-old while waiting for the doctor? Blow up a latex glove (provided no one has allergies to it) and play catch!

later that day...

Izzy's fever is gone now, though she's still slightly congested. Her pediatrician has told me the cough will take some time to clear up. Her lungs are clear, ears are fine and she's on the mend. "It just needs to run its course." Better that way. Glad to hear it's treatable with lemon water, honey and elderberry rather than a prescription.

Thursday - May 15, 2014

Fresh country air breathes new life into my spirit, no matter how severely nauseous the medicine makes me. Waking to bird song, just outside my bedroom window, reminds me of Divine presence in my life. Back porch bathing in sunlight fills my heart with gratitude. Can't stay out in it for long these days, because of chemo, but every minute I do feels like heaven or freedom or like I'm finally not sick anymore.

Doctors told me I was "technically" cancer free after surgery last December. Chemo was a preventative measure, in case they missed anything during surgery. There was hemorrhaging and weight loss when I had cancer but cancer never made me feel half as sick as chemo does.

Cancer weakened my physical state then chemo came along to tear down my psyche through exhaustion, neuropathy, insomnia, chronic constipation, depression and fatigue. Let's not forget hair loss, bleeding gums, a weakened immune system and mood swings. Makes you want to avoid mirrors altogether.

This moment, with Izzy playing on the deck while I journal from the comfort of a cozy patio chair, is all that matters. Warm sunshine kisses my face. Cool breezes hug my skin. This is God's grace. A moment of peace in the storm.

Friday - May 16, 2014

A friend of mine stopped by with a few scaly friends of his own for Dom and Izzy to hang out with. His reptile business visits schools and homes alike promoting awareness about the cold-blooded compadres he looks after. He's pretty much the "reptile whisperer." We lucked out that he was in the next town over, just finishing up one of his programs.

Izzy wasn't the least bit scared of a massive Python that took both Dom and my friend to transport back to its carrier. There was also a toad as big as her head and a large bearded dragon.

I was reminded today to keep the wonder within me alive. To have fun. To not shit my pants when a snake, that can swallow my two-year-old whole, is slithering across the grass. But mostly to continue seeing the world around me with a state of gratitude and awe.

There's a bird of some kind who loves perching atop the roof of the house. When he whistles I whistle back, then he flies up and does a dance only to fly back down to his perch. Our conversations have been going on for about a week now and it's the sweetest thing.

Red breasted house finches nest just outside my bedroom window. They wake me with the sweetest of bird songs. Wild bunnies have made an appearance. It will officially feel like summer, though, when the dragonflies return.

On days when I can't get out of bed, all I need do is open my window to feel close to nature.

Monday - May 19, 2014

Epic adventure today! Traveled to Concord, Massachusetts with a classmate from the *Travel Writing in Sicily* class. We sat at the edge of Walden Pond dipping our toes in history. We sauntered through the very same woods as Henry David Thoreau, walked around his bean garden. Explored a replica of his cabin. Perfect weather for it too. Felt surreal to walk the very same paths as one of my favorite authors. Pure magic.

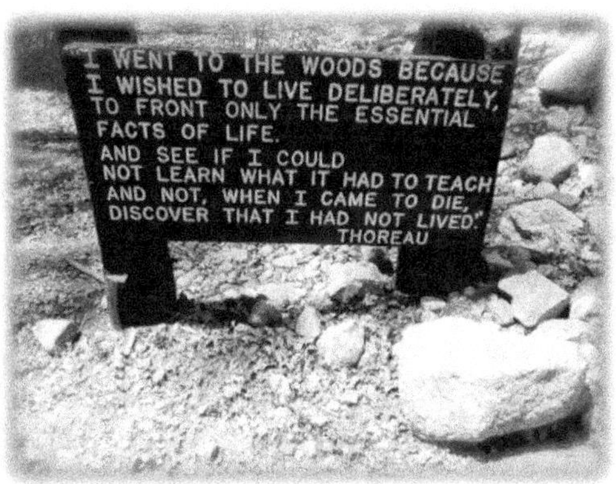

Tuesday - May 20, 2014
CHEMO SESSION # 6

Had this bizarre dream I was in the movie *Fight Club*. Not surprising since Izzy woke me up with a kick to the face and an accidental head-butt to my ribs. Thank you restless little one, for climbing into my bed and kicking my ass in your sleep! So much for being well rested before chemo.

Completed session six today. Ugh...

On the upside, I'm half way through treatments. Only six more to go. *Six.* Sounds like a lifetime.

Most exhausting dose of treatment I've gone through yet. Fatigue overtook my body before the session was half way through. All I thought about was resting, sleep, my queen size bed. I wanted to crawl out of my own skin from the feeling treatment left me with. Sleep was my only option. Usually it takes at least a few hours, sometimes a day, before I feel run down. Today's session hit me hard before I ever left the hospital.

Mom accompanied me for treatment, as she thankfully always does. No way I was driving when we left. I fell asleep in the car on our ride home, only a short twenty-minute drive away. Didn't say a word

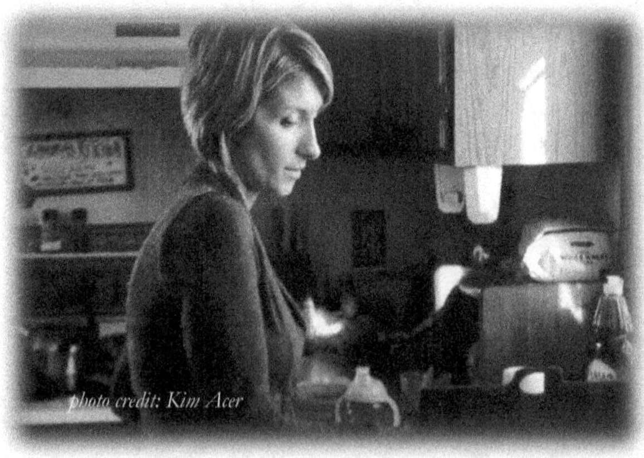

upon waking. My bed was calling out to me; plush pillows, comfy mattress, snuggly blanket.

Off to bed I went to bed; a "mombie" slowly slumping along, not nearly quick enough, toward my temporary resting place. It was close to 3 p.m. by the time we arrived home. Dom would be getting off the bus soon and Izzy would need to be picked up from preschool. I was in no condition to do either.

Mom came into my room. She found me wrapped in a cocoon of blankets, sheets and throw pillows. "Do you want me to call out of work today kiddo? I can get Dom off the bus for you and pick up Izzy. Your father is on his way over to take Dom to baseball practice. I can take Iz to the park and let you get some rest. You have to let me know if you need me to stay home."

Maybe it's the feeling of wanting to maintain control over *something* in my life after feeling totally powerless. Maybe it comes down to pride. I've raised Dom and Iz on my own for so long. Independence is something I've fought long and hard to regain. Kills me emotionally to ask anyone else for help. I'd prefer if she didn't miss a single day of work because of me.

Even "Wonder Woman" has to rest sometimes. After a brief hesitation, I told Mom, *Yes, I need you both today.* Trying to sleep with all these steroids pumping through my veins is impossible, but I'm going to try. Mom is running out of days she can take off at work. I have to take advantage of her help today. My heart is pounding so heavy it feels like it's about to break through my sternum.

Wednesday - May 21, 2014

Slept from 3 p.m. yesterday afternoon until nearly 8 p.m. last night. Woke up for a few hours then went right back to bed until seven this morning. Felt energized, ready to take on the day. Packed up Dom's snack for school, let him and Izzy sleep in a bit and got their things together for the day.

That's when I noticed a few drops of clear liquid on my arm. There were a few more drops on the countertop next to me. *Water must have splashed on the counter when I washed my hands,* I thought to myself. I grabbed a paper towel, quickly wiped up the spill and went into the bathroom to brush my teeth.

More red droplets in the bathroom. On the counter, a few on the floor. I tracked the trail of droplets back into the kitchen. I looked down to notice my shirt was slightly soiled. *There must be a leak somewhere in my chemo pump.*

After initial in-house chemo, I'm given a forty-eight-hour take home pump. It fits into a black fanny pack type of bag that I can either drape over my shoulder like a purse or wear about my waist like an actual fanny pack. The base of the pump is a small box-like structure kept secure within the "fanny pack."

There's a cartridge for the chemotherapy agents that goes into the base. Extending from the cartridge is a long line of tubing.

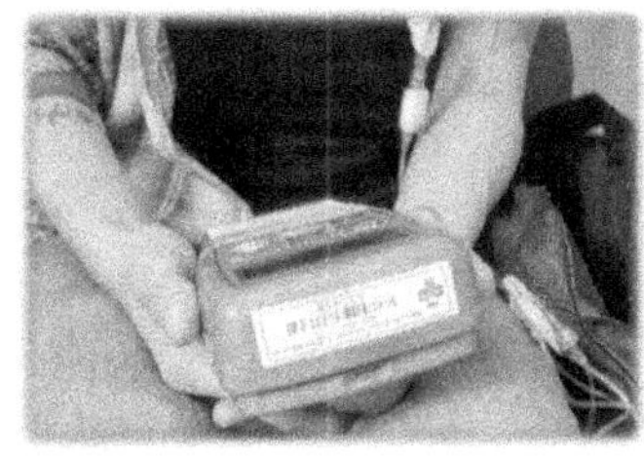

The tubing itself isn't that thick around, the diameter being maybe one centimeter. At the end of that tubing is a screw top that fits into the screw top portion of another line of tubing. That second line of tubing is what connects to the needle inserted into my port.

I checked the tubing connected to the IV needle in my port. It was okay. I followed the line down to where the port tube connects to the chemo tube. Shit! The tubing had come apart.

The red droplets were my blood. Blood and chemotherapy agents were leaking all over the bathroom, the kitchen and me.

My nurse had wrapped tape around the screw caps once they were fastened to ensure leak-free tubing, but for whatever reason the tubing separated.

What do I do now? Stop the leak. I clamped off both lines of the chemo tubes, then wrapped paper towels around the ends that had been leaking. *Okay, got that taken care of. Crap, the bus will be here soon and I haven't woken up Dom yet.*

It was time to wake up Mom! She jumped out of bed, woke up both kiddos, made them breakfast and helped me gather the rest of their things for school. I frantically raced about the house, calling the oncology department to find out what to do next. Fortunately, the infusion suite was open. The nurse on the phone told me to come in as soon as I could to let them take a look at everything.

Dom missed the bus. Mom and me dropped him off at school, then brought Izzy to preschool before we popped in to the hospital. The nurses of the infusion suite were as baffled as I was that the tubing had separated. The needle didn't need replacing, just the tubing and the bag of chemo.

Thursday - May 22, 2014

Been up since 4:30 am! *Thing 1* climbed into bed with me at which point *Thing 2* whispered "Mommy, I want some peanut butter toast on a bagel please." Hoped she would go back to sleep. Until I heard "and apple juice Mommy, I want some apple juice in my sippy. Mommy, apple juice please."

Izzy *(Thing 2)* had her snack, I made banana bread from scratch and little miss is now cooking me eggs in her play kitchen. "Almost done Mommy, at fifty o'clock okay? It's not done yet. You want some eggs too Mommy? Okay, I'll make eggs for you."

After yesterdays' chemo pump mishap, waking up with this little lady is exactly what the doctor ordered.

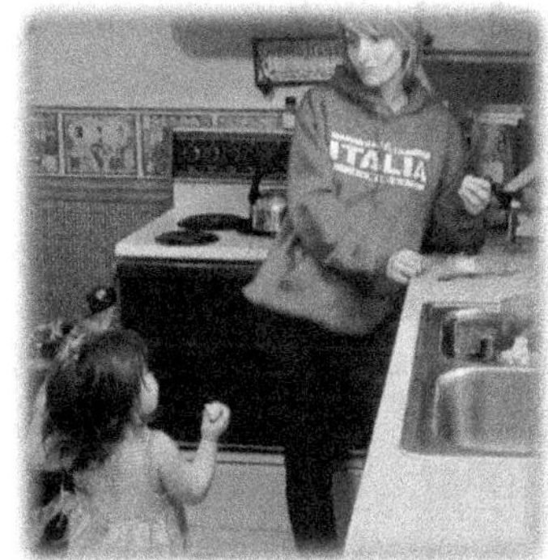

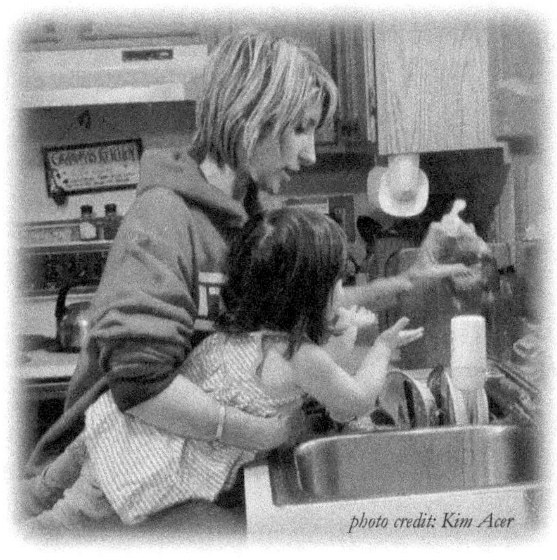

photo credit: Kim Acer

Saturday - May 24, 2014

Ended up having to wear my chemo pack a few hours longer than expected this week. The hours lost to a leaking pump had to be made up. I have to be ready for anything when it comes to chemo. Not only the side effects but the rare occurrence of a malfunctioning piece of equipment. I'm learning to take each treatment it as it comes. Deal with it in stride and take it one day at a time.

Much needed road trip today with *Buddha* for a seminar in Boston. I've been looking forward to it for months. I can already hear the "So Buddha and Super Woman walk into a seminar" jokes coming on. It's going to be a better weekend for sure.

7
JUNE 2014
Release & Allow

> *"Stop trying to control your life, it gets in the way of divine intervention."*
> ~*Cheryl Richardson*

Tuesday - June 3, 2014
CHEMO SESSION # 7
weight: 127.6 pounds/57.87 kilograms

It's amazing how one person's energy can turn your whole day around for the better simply by being them self. Came down with a case of the "grumpies" at infusion this morning, wishing chemo was over and done with. Then my favorite nurse came in and I'm already feeling my mood lift and shift toward being myself again. *Thanks Universe, you've pleasantly surprised me yet again.*

Today I am especially thankful for Kim, for always being
there for me and feeding my starving belly when I've forgotten to eat breakfast because I was in such a rush. Found myself in tears of joy thinking about the close friends and family who have supported me

through chemo, this whole journey really, since being diagnosed.

My family rescued me from emotional turmoil today, without even knowing their kindness was needed. Love, faith, family; these are the greatest riches anyone could ask for.

Wednesday - June 4, 2014

Loving what working out at the gym is doing for me emotionally and physically. Endorphins are flowing baby! Nothing like a great workout to make chemo a hell of a lot easier to go through.

Friday - June 6, 2014
{*Izzy's Birthday*}

"If you ever want to give up, just remember,
there is a little girl watching who wants to be just like you.
Don't disappoint her."
~unknown

Three years ago today, a little love came into my life, opening my heart in a big way. Never imagined being able to love another child as much as I love Dom. When Izzy was born all of that changed. How surprising it was to me, the way she wrapped me

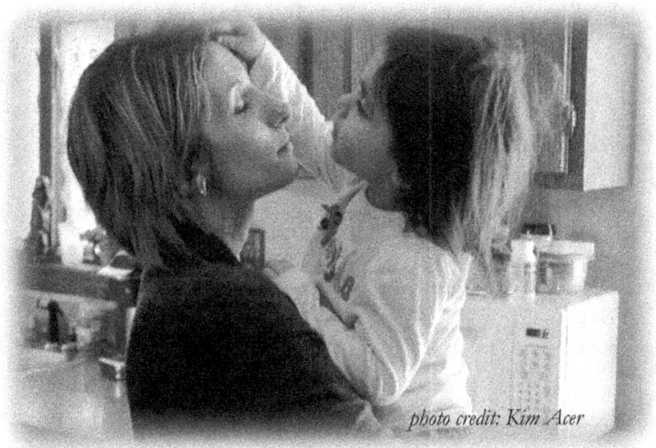

photo credit: Kim Acer

around her finger from the moment of her first breath.

Her personality captivates me now; fiery, fierce yet full of love. She inspires me to be the best version of me because I know even when I'm not looking, she's watching me.

It wasn't long after I started wearing a chemo pump home that Izzy started wearing her purses off to the side just like her Mom. She'd tell me, "See Mommy, I have a chemo pump just like you." Am I to feel proud that she admires me so? Am I to feel saddened because she doesn't realize Mommy's chemo pouch isn't a purse?   Izzy is far too young to understand the depth of the situation. She's experienced me having good days, when my spirit is full of energy. She's also seen the days when Grandma has to get her ready for school or pick her up because "Mommy is too tired." When I can't get out of bed, she climbs in next to me to snuggle. She uplifts my spirits with her laughter, lends me her strength when I am at my weakest. Happy Birthday fierce little one. Thank you for being part of the strength that carries me through.

Friday - June 13, 2014

Michael Franti playing in the background, adding a bit of Feng Shui to my sanctuary, saging my space to raise the good vibrations! Feeling healthy, strong and blessed. Today is a good day.

Sunday - June 15, 2014

Over the last six months Dad has been an inspirational part of my life. He's been cooking, doing dishes, taking Dom to every one of his baseball practices and games, even entertaining Izzy with her games and dolls.

When I haven't the strength to get out of bed, Dad looks after Dom and Iz without hesitating.

He's been "stopping by to say hello" so he tells me, when he's "in the area." *Just so you know Dad,* I think to myself, *I totally know you weren't in the area.* It's been pretty "convenient" that he seems to be nearby during treatment week.

Pretty sure there's some type of collaboration effort between him and Mom going on. Some days I'm just getting off the phone with Mom, when Dad calls in or vice versa. This journey has been a challenging one. Yet I can

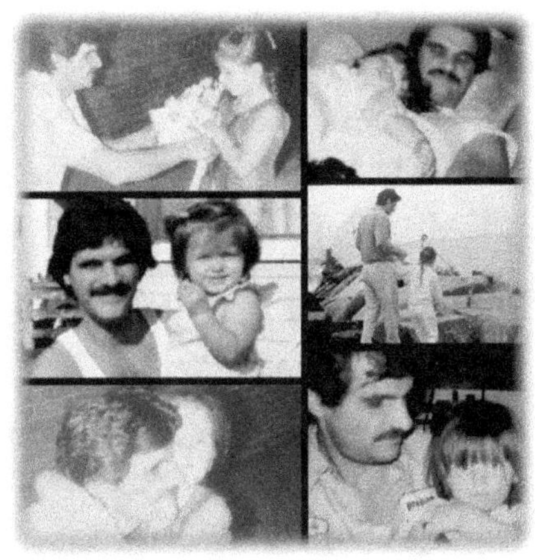

honestly say I am thankful because I've never been as close to either one of my parents as I am now. I am thankful for them, thankful for this journey.

Dad is not only pulling for me; he's pulling me through this. He's been so gracious with his time, especially for a man who isn't exactly known for his patience. The gratitude I have for that man is boundless.

Happy Father's Day Dad. You are loved. You are appreciated.

Tuesday - June 17, 2014

Today's mantra: "My body and my thoughts are stronger than chemo or cancer. I AM a survivor and I can do this, with the love and support of my family. The Universe is constantly taking care of me."

Scheduled for chemo session number eight but, thank God, there was an angel...or two...or three on my shoulder. The nurse double checked my platelet count before administering meds. Yesterday, the nursing manager missed my platelet count when she checked my file. They're too low for treatment today. I could have bled out internally if they gave me chemo.

Session eight has been canceled.

Tuesday - June 24, 2014
CHEMO SESSION # 8

Four more to go after this! I've got my lavender eye pillow courtesy of "Saint Patrick," stress relief oil from Dom's Godmother, an angel meditation cd from *Buddha* and my personal bodyguard (my brother Nate) to keep me company.

Hoping to Zen myself out during chemo. Good vibes only.

Friday - June 27, 2014

Feeling a little under the weather today, but doing what I can to stay focused and not let these chemo side effects get the best of me. Got to focus on the positive.

Izzy woke up in such a great mood, she put an instant smile on my face. Missing Dom while he's away with Felipe's side of the family. Judging from the pictures they've sent, he's having an amazing time.

Saturday - June 28, 2014

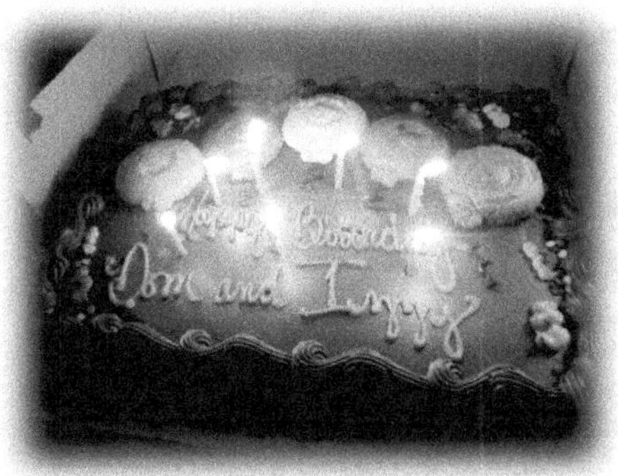

It's been hard financially this year. I was talking to my sister, Kim, about the kids the other day. Dom turned eight this year and Izzy turned three. They both asked for a birthday party but it wasn't within my means to provide either one of them with one. Kim listened contently, all the while the gears in her head were already turning.

"What about a joined birthday party? We can have it at my house. I'll take care of everything." The thing about my sister, is that she isn't one of those people who says kind things with no intention of following through. By the time she's mentioned her idea, she's already gone through a brief rundown of the logistics in her head. This time was no exception.

Kim took care of the cake, party supplies, snacks for the kids and all of the details. I provided burgers, hot dogs, buns and the drinks. There were games to play and cousins to play them with. More food than we could all eat. She took time out of her busy life to be there for Dom, Izzy and me. She thoughtfully planned every detail, creating a worry free celebration for their birthdays.

Monday - June 30, 2014

Much too tired to write for long. Stayed up until nearly five in the morning, binge watching *Scandal* on Netflix with Nate. We don't get to spend nearly as much time together since we live so far away from one another.

Scandal is such an addicting show! Staying up all night, giving each-other the "you want to watch another episode?" look after each one ended. We could have watched more but it would have required taping our eyelids open. When we lived together, we'd stay up until all hours of the night watching movies and shows together on the weekend. I miss it. I miss spending time with him.

Except for that one night we stayed up watching *The Ring*. We shut all the lights off after the movie to head upstairs to our rooms. He was walking behind me in the dark and began making that freaky, creaking noise from the movie. I've never ran up those damn stairs faster than I did that night! I miss his practical jokes too. Even though we stayed up so late, I'm feeling recharged today. Needed that family time with my big bro, long overdue.

Izzy has been quite funny today. I let out a long sigh about something. Izzy walks over to me, says "Mommy, I'm going to kiss you, then you don't say 'huhhhh' no more okay?" The kisses she left on my cheek over and over had me laughing so hard. Mostly because of the intense duck face she made while doing it.

A moment ago she was painting outside on the deck when her paper flew away. She looked out into the sky shouting "Shiver me timbers! It's very windy today!" There are countless blessings within a day, if we're open to receiving them.

8
JULY 2014
Gratitude

"If the only prayer you ever say in your entire life is 'thank you,'
it will be enough.
~Meister Eckhart

Wednesday - July 2, 2014

Five days away from 30! Still feel like I'm in my early twenties. So good to be entering my thirties free of emotional baggage. Thank you, cancer, for helping me step onto a path of healing. I'm moving forward in every aspect of my life, moving toward perfect health and almost done with treatments!

Friday - July 4, 2014

Izzy was phenomenal today during her first plane ride! Dom had flown countless times by the time he was her age. I was worried she might be scared but my little daredevil loved it! I'm elated to be spending the next week with my brother and my nephew. A week in the Florida sunshine will do us all some good; me, Mom, Izzy. It's been a long year. Mom and me have certainly earned ourselves a vacation.

Nate took us all out to *Jacksonville Landing* tonight. We celebrated Independence Day, together as a family, watching fireworks go off over the water. My heart is full.

Monday - July 7, 2014

Happy Birthday to me! Today is my 30th birthday. Most would say turning thirty doesn't feel different - it does for me. Last December my surgeon told me if I had waited another six months to be seen, there would have been nothing they could do for me. Yet here I am! Thankful for the gift of life.

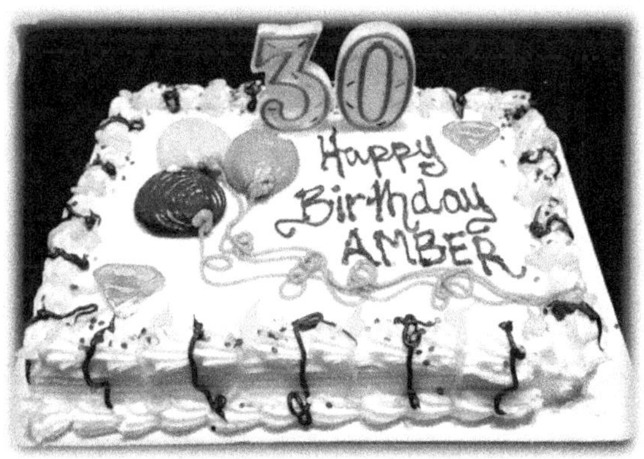

Friday - July 11, 2014

Home cooked meal at Nate's for our farewell dinner together as a family. He's made bruschetta, chicken parmesan and baked pasta with cheese and sauce. If he spoiled us like this the entire trip, we'd never leave. Maybe that's why he waited until tonight.

Monday - July 14, 2014

No chemo tomorrow, white cells too low.

Tuesday - July 15, 2014

My side effects have been minimal in comparison to other patients undergoing the same treatment. Why? Is it age? Does it have to do with cultivating a state of gratitude on a daily basis? Is it exercise? Eating healthy? I don't know for certain what has helped me move through this trial with what others have called "grace."

I know I have shit days just like anyone else. When I feel awful, I sit with it. But I don't choose to "live" there.

I've found when sitting with sadness or hopelessness - gratitude acts as a lifeline pulling me out. It's pretty damn hard to maintain an emotional state of sheer misery when I'm looking at the dimples in my daughter's hands. I can't be angry or sad or depressed when I see Dom look at Izzy with admiration and love, in spite of thinking he's "way too cool" to hang out with her anymore.

Thinking of the many cancer patients out there, right now, struggling to survive brings me to a tearful place of reality. I've experienced severe side effects but was given a hopeful prognosis with a high chance of remission.

I think of my Aunt Anne, battling the late stages of lung cancer for years. Going to chemo alone. Not really having anyone to reach out to because she's been so disconnected from the family for so long. I think of the patients who have grown tired of treatment, experienced countless surgeries, bloodwork and hospitalizations. The ones tired of not being able to live their best life because of a constant state of dis-ease in their body.

My heart is with them on a daily basis. I wish I could sit with every one of them, hold their hand, tell them "you're not alone." I wish I could be there for the cancer patients who don't have anyone to turn to.

I want to be there to assure them they can still take back some level of control from cancer. Even if they don't have anyone else to lean on, they can still search within themselves to tap into their own personal power. We all have the ability to do it. Even us cancer patients. *Especially* us cancer patients, in my opinion.

While the doctors prescribed medications to treat my body, I found ways of empowering myself and uplifting my spirit. Reiki, meditation, constant prayers of gratitude, exercise and channeling positive emotion through music have all saved my life.

This past Saturday I attended a Dave Matthews Band concert for the first time. Between the music and the band's stage presence, the concert was absolutely phenomenal. It got me thinking about some of my favorite songs. Whether they are new age, hard rock, EDM, Motown, classical, etc. I thought of how those songs make me feel. Thought about their power to elevate my mood from a state of stagnancy to a hip-swaying, feel good euphoria.

There have been numerous studies on how music affects the brain from how our bodies respond during exercise[1,2] to productivity and mood elevation[3]. Music has been shown to affect the cognitive learning ability of children for the better[4]. It has been scientifically proven to help the human body soothe away stress as well[5].

When I'm feeling exhausted, not in the best place emotionally, too tired to go to the gym – I have a "go to" playlist of songs. They breathe life into my lungs and make my heart beat steady again. They get me off of the couch to dance with my children, channeling the silliest moves my body can make. These songs make me smile, make me laugh but most of all elicit a type of soul awakening joy.

If every cancer patient could find just one song that makes them feel that way, even if for a brief moment, the world would seem brighter. Find it, feel it, close your eyes and breathe life in.

Kicking Cancer's Ass playlist

- Michael Franti, *I'm Alive*
- Michael Franti, *Sound of Sunshine*
- Colbie Caillat, *Brighter Than the Sun*
- Cupid, *Cupid Shuffle*
- One Republic, *Marchin' On*
- Bob Marley, *Three Little Birds*
- Queen, *We Will Rock You*
- Imagine Dragons, *On Top of the World*
- War, *Low Rider*
- The White Stripes, *Seven Nation Army*
- Matisyahu, *One Day*
- Imagine Dragons *Ready Aim Fire*
- V.I.C., *Wobble*

Wednesday - July 16, 2014

Just got in from a regular checkup with my primary care doctor. Blood pressure, weight, reflexes, etc. are all within normal range. My doctor was amazed at how well I look since going through chemo. He said he'd never be able to tell I'm going through what I am physically if he didn't already know. Feeling fabulous!

Saturday - July 19, 2014

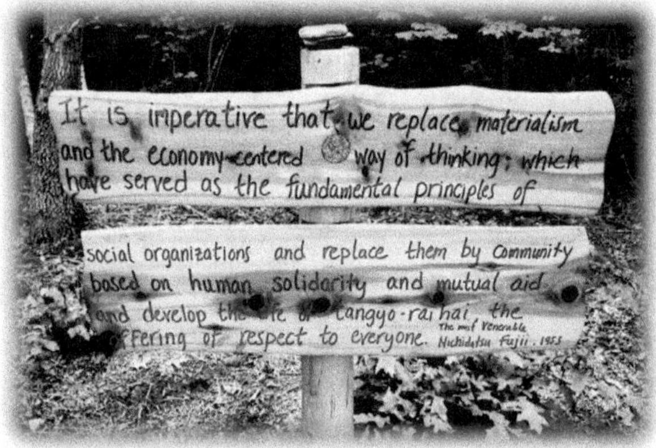

Visited the *Peace Pagoda* today with *Buddha*. Frogs swam in the pond, surfacing only to drink in air. Waterlilies floated above them, unshaken by the movement of frog or Koi below. Dragonflies danced all around us. Much magic there to be breathed in by the senses. Beauty all around in the simplest of moments.

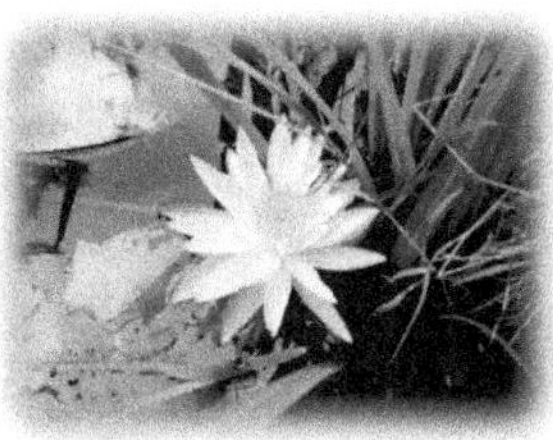

Tuesday - July 22, 2014
CHEMO SESSION # 9

After today, I have three treatments left. Not five or six or eleven, just three.

It's quite beautiful outside. The sun offers warmth as it shines the narrow window of my infusion suite. People are visible out in the hospital parking lot; parking cars, running into neighboring buildings for appointments, picking up loved ones. A world of strangers oblivious to the dozen or so of us currently receiving treatment.

The words of Michael Franti's song *The Sound of Sunshine* are replaying in my mind. When I listen to that song, it doesn't matter how low my mental or emotional state is. The sound of his voice and the rhythm of the instruments playing in the background uplifts my spirit to a sacred space of joy. Happiness. Health.

His music makes me feel like I'm not sitting here in my chemo chair receiving treatment. I close my eyes, letting the chorus transport me; *I'm on the beach getting sand in my toes and some other less desirable places. Dom and Izzy are there. My siblings, my parents and my nieces and nephews are too. We're cooking on the grill, watching all of our babes splash around in the waves. The smell of barbecue chicken fills my senses.*

There are so many ways to pass the time during chemo; sleep, read, watch movies, write, play cards, chat with someone. My vices today shall be music and writing.

I'm happy to be here today, thankful there are only three treatments in my future after this. I'm grateful it was caught early enough to treat.

There's an elderly gentleman here receiving treatment. He looks to be in his sixties, possibly seventies. He and his wife are seated diagonally across from me to the left. I can't take my eyes off them. It's lunch time. All of the chemo patients have been served our lunches, save for me. My Superstar sister, Kim, brought me lunch today.

The elderly gentleman looks to be a tall man if he were standing. His petite wife stands beside him, roughly the same height while he is sitting. I imagine his stature would tower over her if they stood next to one another.

She delicately feeds him small bites of the sandwich he's ordered. Every so often, she gives him a small spoonful of soup, perhaps to help the sandwich go down easier. He doesn't seem fully capable of feeding himself.

His wife walks away to grab a few napkins for her spouse. The gentleman looks over his lunch tray in her absence. His hand passes over each item on the tray; strawberry layer cake, a Styrofoam cup of soup, his sandwich. His hand passes over the food like an audience member asked to "pick a card, any card" by a magician.

His wife returns with a hand full of napkins, ready to lovingly dab away any excess crumbs or spilled soup from his chin. Her compassionate love for him is apparent with every gentle wipe of his face, each spoonful of soup she nourishes him with. Her fragile hands hold the bendy straw of his drink with such grace and love as she lifts it to his lips.

Watching their interactions, as I write this, brings tears to my eyes. Anyone else would have probably walked past without even noticing. Yet, I sit here pondering how anyone could witness such an intimate moment of vulnerability and not tear up. Their love is beautiful. Kind. Eloquent. The type of love we should all count ourselves fortunate to have, if we are lucky enough to find it.

9
AUGUST 2014
Strength

*"The strength of a woman is not measured by the impact that
all her hardships in life have had on her; but the strength of a
woman is measured by the extent of her refusal to allow those
hardships to dictate her and who she becomes."*
~C. Joybell C.

Tuesday - August 5, 2014
CHEMO SESSION # 10

*"For He will command his angels concerning you to guard you
in all your ways."*
~Psalm 91:11

Only two more chemo sessions to go after today!!! In the beginning I felt like this would never end. Now I'm almost done and on the road to my survivorship! Woot woot!

Feeling thankful today and every day. Looking forward to getting my chemo pump off so I can get back in the gym in a few days.

Tuesday - August 12, 2014

Chemo has reduced by voluminous thick locks to paper thin sections of hair. No one seems to notice but me. I've decided to go with a short, sassy pixie cut in case it all falls before treatment is finished.

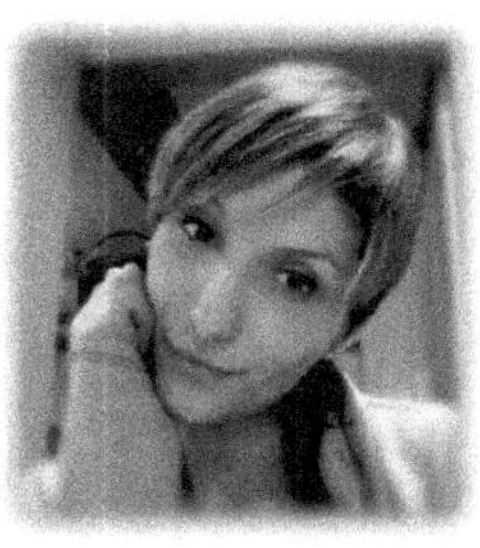

Still can't get over Robin Williams passing. I'll never forget his performance in *Awakenings* with Robert DeNiro or the inescapable tears *What Dreams May Come* evokes. Williams left behind a legacy of tears and laughter. I grew up watching *Mork and Mindy* on *Nick at Night*. When my siblings weren't around I'd try to drinking water from a glass by dipping my finger in it, just like Mork. The world has lost a profound human being. Might watch *Hook* with Dom later on. I could use a bit of laughter.

Going through chemo while trying to keep track of baseball games and practices for Dom, waking up early for Saturday morning gymnastics with Izzy, chauffeuring Dom to martial arts training, attending school functions, play dates and birthday parties - has been excruciatingly exhausting. That doesn't take into account my own classes, homework or doctor appointments. I never gave too much thought to it. Took it on, am still doing it, one day at a time.

People have told me how strong they think I am. Brave. Courageous. One tough cookie. They've said they're proud of me for moving along the journey with such positivity.

The truth is, when you're going through something like this, you do what has to be done. Sure there's moments of doubt. Moments of wanting to quit chemo. Moments of thinking, *screw this, I'd rather be at home spending time with my kids than in the hospital getting more blood work or another infusion.*

Those moments come in briefly. I acknowledge them, honor what I'm feeling, then move on. Life is too short. Too precious to be wasted on negative thoughts, negative energy. Regardless of what anyone feels or thinks, that clock of life keeps ticking away. I'd rather spend my days surrounded by the ones I love, helping others, raising my children to be genuinely decent human beings. Giving love, embracing forgiveness, moving to the beat of my own drum in tune with the rhythm of life.

Going back to being labeled as strong…

When I hear people say how strong I am, it doesn't quite register. Aren't we *all* strong in one way or another? Some of us are emotionally strong, others physically or intellectually. There's countless ways for a person to be *strong.*

We *all* have greatness within us. We're all sparks of divine creation. Seriously. It's not accidental that any of us are here. If we're alive and our hearts are beating, we need to be thankful because we hit the ultimate lottery. If that sperm had fertilized a different egg or different swimmer won the race, I wouldn't be sitting here writing about it in my journal. I wouldn't be me.

No one knows what it's like to actually go through this. No one but those of us in the cancer community. My mother knows what it's like to see me in a state of complete exhaustion. My father knows what it's like to be there for my children when I'm too nauseous, feeling too sick to function. My siblings know what it's like to watch me connected to an intravenous line of medication, sitting in the infusion suite for hours on end until treatment is done. Only a cancer patient knows ALL of the ups and downs. The things we keep hidden from family members to prevent them from worrying more than usual.

I don't see myself as this brave woman going through cancer treatment. A fighter, yes. A woman doing what she has to do to survive, absolutely. I'm doing what I have to so my children and I can live our best life, expand and thrive. They're going to have memories of mom wearing that chemo pump for days at a time. Memories of having to get popsicles, ice cream or frozen yogurt pops out of the open freezer because it literally caused me pain to go near it.

Maybe not Izzy so much but Dom will remember all of it.

They're also going to have memories of family gatherings and barbecues. Memories of visits with their grandparents and uncle out of state, going to Florida on vacation, playing *Dance Dance Revolution* for hours on the Wii at their Auntie's house with me, summer fun festivals and dance off competitions. Izzy will remember *Mommy and Me* gymnastics, playtime at the park and snuggles before bed. Dom will revisit movie night madness memories, remember fishing with Grandpa.

I'll have memories as well, beyond dis-ease. Memories of Dom leaving a gentle, quiet kiss on my forehead as I rested on the couch. Or covering me with a blanket because he thought I was sleeping. The times Izzy snuck in my room to give me a quick snuggle before Grandma caught her interrupting my rest. Their laughter, their jokes. God, even the arguments and attitude will be looked back on with fondness. Because I witnessed it all first hand. I was there with them every step of the way.

Our lives have all changed in some way since my diagnosis. The *quality* of my children's lives, of my life, has only gotten better. It took a life-threatening diagnosis for me to prioritize what matters. Cancer became more than dis-ease in my body. As trying as it's been, cancer turned out to be my cure. It's given me the power to focus on gratitude toward the healthy relationships in my life, releasing the unhealthy ones.

Cancer broke my heart open. Let the healing in. Like a "secret treasure" as Izzy would say, there was hidden strength locked away within the depths of my soul. Cancer just pushed me to find it.

So do I have a great deal of strength within me now from all of this? Most definitely. Do I consider myself a strong person? I suppose. Mostly though? I see myself as stubborn, resilient and unwilling to let cancer take control of my life.

I see strength in the eyes of my mother, every time she has to drive me to chemo. The hope that these treatments are working. The pain of her having to watch me go through all of this. It's hit her harder than anyone, harder than me. That woman

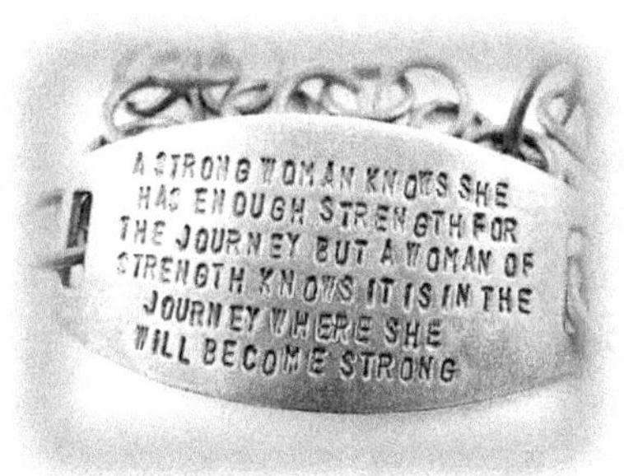

has unrelenting strength and I love her so much for it.

The strength to care for two small children after working forty plus hour work weeks; all so I can rest. The strength to watch the transformation every treatment week as my energy is zapped away for two or three days or more.

The people around me, surrounding me with love and healing energy, those are the strong ones. The people who silently stand by me, unable to "fix" me or do anything other than offer emotional support.

That's strength. Watching someone you care about go through a cancer battle. Being selfless enough to care for them. To stay with them emotionally, not everyone can handle that. I'm thankful for the people in my life who can. I'm thankful, as well, to have become strong enough to let go of the ones who can't.

If I could share what I've learned with other cancer patients, I would say;

Take everything one day at a time. Focus on the positive. Focus on the good in your life. Know that there is a power within you able to see you through anything. No matter how shitty your day is, gratitude can always be found if we don't blind ourselves to it. Don't take anything for granted, including yourself.

Perseverance of the human spirit in the face of adversity is a powerful thing. Don't give up on yourself. Count your blessings twice. None of us know for certain what the future brings but while you're still here, why not make this life the best life you can?

Thursday - August 14, 2014

Tomorrow I'm going in for a quick office procedure, just to check things out, had a bit of a scare today. My doctor feels that everything will be fine but I just need the peace of mind. My mind is racing. What if the cancer comes back? What if chemo isn't working?

When I look back on my life, I want to remember all of the good that was in it. All of the people I loved and who loved me in return, every person who was there when I was at my best and pulled me through the pain when I was at my worst.

Friday - August 15, 2014

My office exam went extremely well today. There's minor irritation around my internal staples but other than that everything looks really good. I'm okay!

Thankful for having the time and energy to cook a big, family, sit-down dinner two nights in a row.

Monday - August 18, 2014

Dom starts third grade in about a week and a half. Third grade! Blessed to be his Mama. Where has the time gone?

Speaking of time. It's been nearly two weeks since my last chemo session but the side effects are lingering. Woke up this morning feeling extremely unwell. It wasn't so much my mental state as it was my physical body. Getting out of bed sounded horrible. The nausea was unbearable. Didn't want to eat a damn thing or even think about food.

Canceled chemo tomorrow because I'm getting Level II Reiki certified this weekend. Detoxing the body is an important part of Reiki attunement preparation. Being injected with chemo agents didn't seem like the greatest idea. Hope I'm feeling better by Friday. Usually when my physical state starts dipping, my mental state isn't far behind. I was having thoughts of giving up on treatment again. *Do I really need to finish? It's only two treatments.*

After a few hours of feeling sorry for myself, I decided it was time to get my shit together. *Okay, Amber,* I told myself, *pull yourself out of this. Go online, find some guided gratitude mediations. Inspirational speeches. Anything to pick your spirits up. Do something.*

I went online and started searching for gratitude videos. That didn't work. I changed my search to "videos about being a strong woman." On the side bar of the website there was a recommended video about confidence and mindsets that drive men wild. I could care less about the "driving men wild" part right now, but something about the guy in the video grabbed my attention and I needed a confidence boost so I clicked on it.

That video enticed me into watching another one about strong women myths. I was about to go back to searching for gratitude meditations after watching the second one when another of his videos popped up. It was a video distinguishing the difference between a person who has quirks and someone who is a good old fashioned nutcase. This one, I *have* to watch.

That third video was the one that got me. I wasn't feeling so bad anymore. Laughter roared from my belly. Nearly started to cough I was laughing so hard. I spent the next few hours watching his videos. Through satire, logic and his ability to be unapologetically himself – those videos pulled me out of what was becoming a deep state of depression.

He's got some type of women's retreat he runs too. It supposedly takes clients through ten years of growth over the course of one week. Looks interesting enough. Should be hearing from someone at his company soon since I just reached out to request more info.

Tuesday - August 19, 2014

Spoke with someone from that company about the retreat today. She's sending me an application for the program and then once I send it back to her, we'll set up a phone interview to go over it and see if I'm ready for the retreat.

I'm feeling apprehensive about applying. I've never heard of this guy or his company before. Could just be another internet scam. We'll see.

Saturday - August 23, 2014

"Everything is energy and that's all there is to it. Match the frequency of the reality you want and you cannot help but get that reality. It can be no other way. This is not philosophy. This is physics."
~Albert Einstein

Completed Reiki level II training this weekend! Already looking forward to completing Reiki Master training in the future. Nama-stay-out-of-my-way everyone, this girl is unstoppable!

Thursday - August 28, 2014

Dear Amber:

Success is the only option. Never settle for anything less than extraordinary. You are worth it.

With Love,
the Universe

Wednesday - August 27, 2014

Dom is getting a fresh new haircut today! First day of school tomorrow. Third grade. Holy hell Batman.

Sunday - August 31, 2014

"I would like my life to be a statement of love and compassion - and where it isn't, that's where my work lies."
~Ram Dass

This coming Wednesday is supposed to be treatment number 11 out of 12. Only two more to go! Over the past eight months, I've done more to enhance my life than I would have - had I not been diagnosed with Cancer.

Prior to my diagnosis, I was living a life of *ordinary* means. It wasn't a bad life, just boring. I ate healthy but I wasn't exercising. My yoga practice was consistently inconsistent. I wasn't disciplined even though I enjoyed it. School was exhausting. I wasn't giving myself enough time. I didn't make self-care a priority.

I was perfectly content to live in the complacency of my daily routine. Repeating the same monotonous patterns every day, holding onto the past instead of living for the moment at hand.

This year I began valuing myself as a mother, spiritual being and woman on a core level. The more I've given to myself, the more I have to give to those I love. I've connected with others in the cancer community with compassionate.

I'm not saying my life is rainbows, butterflies and unicorns all the time. This morning I thought for sure my kids were going to tackle one another. It wasn't in a "let's hug it out" kind of way either. My son was upset because I told him to eat breakfast and clean the rest of his room before he went over his friend's house. My daughter has entered the phase of using her adorableness to persuade me, believing that her use of the word "please" automatically means "yes" to whatever she asks for. They're both learning about boundaries and I'm learning about patience.

We shouldn't wait for a life threatening diagnosis to make our lives extraordinary. It's not a matter of luck or fate or coincidence. If we want change to occur in our lives, we have to be willing to make the changes ourselves that facilitate them. Simple as that. Break out of our routines. Do the things we're scared of, without putting ourselves or anyone else in harm's way of course.

Time is a precious commodity that so many take for granted. There's no waiting for opportunity to knock. We have to break down the damn door. Take initiative. Do the things we love. Appreciate the people who are there for us. Forgive and let go of the ones who aren't. Wake each morning with gratitude that we have another day.

Most of us naively walk around with this thought process of "I'm always going to be around. I have time to do that later. It's not going to happen to *me*." I was guilty of it. Then at twenty-nine-years old, BOOM, I was diagnosed with Stage III Colon Cancer with no family history of the disease.

Life happens. It's about *how* we react when shit hits the fan that matters. It's understandable to be upset or down, have emotions that overwhelm us, feel sad or depressed. It's perfectly normal, it makes us human. After a certain point, it's time to brush the dirt off our shoulders, get our asses up off the floor, proclaim to (the Universe, God, ourselves, whoever) that we are stronger than ever before. Throwing pity parties aren't going to do anything but feed more momentum into a negative situation.

I was feeling overwhelmed today at returning to school this semester, vehicle searching, chemo almost but not quite being done, finding the energy to do what I have to for my children. Then my mother gave me the best piece of advice and something clicked. She said, "You're just going to have to do it. Don't think about and just get through it. You've done it before and you'll do it again."

This past Spring, I never questioned what I had to do. I passed both of my classes with A's, found the time and energy to bring my son to Kung Fu twice a week, to take my daughter to Mommy and me gymnastics every Saturday morning, balanced play dates with study nights and housework, began classes three weeks post op from major colon resection surgery and started chemo. If I could do all of that last semester, I knew it was *absolutely* possible to handle everything now. Mom was right.

There is so much light, strength, beauty, compassion and love within each and every one of us if we'd just be willing to tap into it. Struggles build character, give us something to learn from and can knock us to the ground. If we're able to get back up when life knocks us down, that's the real strength. To smile with gratitude after we've been hurt, to laugh in the face of fear, to persevere with a positive attitude;

that right there is better than all the money in the world combined.

10
SEPTEMBER 2014
Grand Finale

"Soon, when all is well,
you're going to look back on this period of your life
and be glad that you never gave up."
~Brittany Burgunder

Monday - September 1, 2014

Chemo has been canceled two weeks in a row because of low blood counts. I feel great during the day but am usually ready for bed by 7 or 8 p.m. Not sure chemo will be happening this week either if I don't get some energy back soon! Maybe I can pay Dom to rub my feet for me. Or not.

Tuesday - September 2, 2014

First day of Fall university classes! Yes! Getting my new car soon. Feeling immeasurable gratitude for everyone who donated to the *Go Fund Me* page I created. Life *is* good!

Family. The people we sometimes take for granted because no matter what, they're stuck with us. Family can be friends that have been there for us when we hadn't the strength to 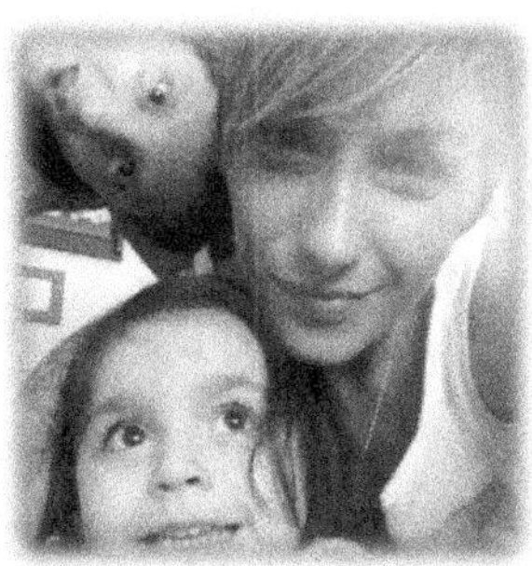 be there for ourselves. People who pull us out of low places. People who tell us what we *need* to hear, not always what we *want* to hear.

Famiglia è tutto, family is everything. A concept ingrained into the very fibers of my DNA, in utero no doubt. Family first, end statement. I thought I'd done a pretty good job of honoring the value of family. It wasn't until diagnosed with cancer, that I realized how disconnected from my family I'd been.

I love them for sure but I didn't really know any of them as well as I knew my own children and we have a super close, super warm family. I began to see my relatives with an open heart of appreciation.

My family has seen me at my moodiest, most exhausted and ornery state of being and continued to love me anyhow. They're emotional soldiers. Onward, they've trudged through the mud of emotional chaos, never once leaving me behind.

I consider the oncology nurses to be my second family. These women are troopers. I overheard one of the other chemo patients talking down to the nurse a bit. His behavior reminded me of my Grandpa Teddy's behavior whenever he was in the hospital; tough as nails and not at all happy about other people being in control of his health. My grandfather's nurses bore the brunt of his attitude problem.

This gentleman was in his mid to late seventies and was no different. "Ya know, I haven't got all day here. I've been waiting almost a half hour. Let's go." He went on about how upset he was and how much he didn't appreciate waiting around for so long. This nurse was exactly the person this man needed to see. She smoothed things out with him, calmed him down and charmed him right out of the funk he was in.

Imagining the number of patients, contrasted personalities, treatment mood swings and everything else in between these nurses deal with from us cancer patients boggles my mind. I know from experience there are treatment days when I don't enjoy being around myself. The nurses should be walking around with superhero capes as far as I'm concerned. Maybe they *do* have capes, they just keep them in a special closet until their shift is over.

I'm going to miss these women when treatment is done. The conversations about our children, or their grandchildren. Fortunate to have so many wonderful people woven into my life. It's created a true structure of emotional stability.

Cancer has changed me for the better. Little things that used to bother me before are easier to let go of. Everyday blessings are welcomed, not looked over with a passing glance. Fully grasping the concept of life's fragility has helped me harness gratitude to the tenth power.

Wednesday - September 3, 2014
CHEMO SESSION # 11

Only one more to go after today, thank you Universe! Mom stayed home from work to take care of me tonight. She cooked one of my favorite recipes. One whiff of her cooking and the nausea was gone. Two bowls later, I was ready for a nap.

She was fabulous to take care of me and the kids like she did. I was able to get to bed early. Unfortunately, I was wired from the steroids so now I'm wide awake. Hoping I can get some rest again after homework, wicked busy day tomorrow. Going to need some sleep.

I've been thinking about my late grandparents today. Grandma Vicki, telling Grandpa to give her the "clicker." No one uses that word for the remote anymore. I miss baking muffins with her. I miss the way she'd hover over me while I mixed the ingredients together. I miss sleepovers at their house, how Grandpa would let me use his "special" pillows. The pillows he never let anyone use. I miss the way Grandma would peer around the corner of her rocking chair to look at me. She'd look over at Grandpa asleep in his chair, then give me the signal to steal the "clicker" from him by raising her eyebrows and nodding her head. As soon as he started to wake up, she'd put on an old black and white wartime movie on so he wouldn't know the difference.

Mom and me were over their house practically every day when she got out of work. Every weekend. We'd have *Fish and Chip Fridays* and coffee and donuts Sunday morning. No coffee for me of course. I made up for it by helping out with the donuts. I was fifteen years old and still asking Mom if I could sleep over their house on the weekends. She was always shocked that her teenage daughter wanted to have sleepovers with her geriatric parents. Seriously? They fed me donuts and muffins for breakfast. They let me stay up all night watching old Hollywood films like, *An Affair to Remember* with Deborah Kerr and Cary Grant or *Cover Girl* with Rita Hayworth and Gene Kelly.

Anytime I want to feel close to my grandparents or find myself missing them terribly, I sit down to watch old Hollywood classics. I fell in love with those movies then and I love them still today.

Thursday - September 4, 2014

This is how chemo and steroids make me feel when I want to sleep; *one sheep, two sheep, three sheep, blue, cow, chicken, duck, Old MacDonald had a farm. Heyyyyyyy macarena!*

Saturday - September 6, 2014

Dom has filled up bottles of water for everyone, brought food down to the basement and has now convinced Izzy to assist him with gathering blankets, pillows and anything else we need for the thunderstorm watch that's in effect. As the "man of the house," he takes his responsibilities seriously. I told him, jokingly, he's been watching too much *Survivor man.*

It poured for all of ten minutes. When the rain stopped, Dom said, "I can't believe I did all that for no reason!" True, but it was extremely entertaining to watch!

Sunday - September 7, 2014

My sis, Kim, participated in a *Mudderella* yesterday and wrote my name on a lantern with a few

others as part
of the course. I
woke up this
morning to
picture
messages from
her and
couldn't stop
crying.

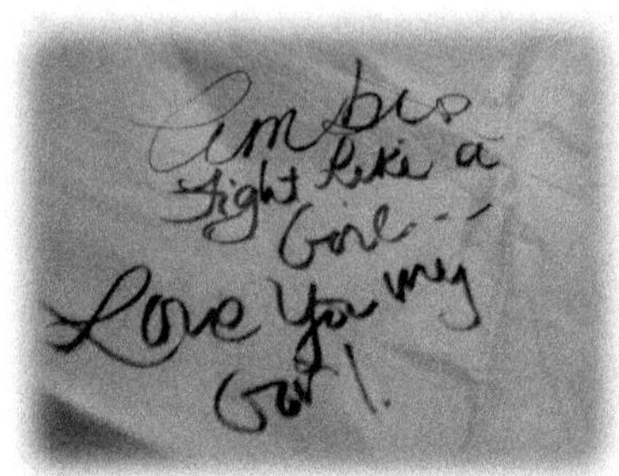

Saturday - September 13, 2014

Dad stopped by. He'd only planned on staying for a quick visit. When he arrived, I didn't have the strength to get up and greet him with my usual bear hug. He took one look at me and asked if I needed him to stay. Without hesitation I told him how much I would appreciate it if he did.

He ended up sleeping over. He watched Izzy until she fell asleep. He watched her again first thing in the morning when she woke up.

I curled up to Dom, watching movies for the rest of the night. He put on *Full House* because he knows I have a crush on John Stamos. He shared his half-inch-tall, rubber, *Trash Pack* collection with me. Crushed soda cans with faces, rotten cheeseburgers with googly eyes. Some of them are actually sort-of cute.

I don't know how I'd get through this journey of cancer without my family. My father has been there for me like I never could have imagined. He's taken Dom to martial arts on several occasions. He brought him to nearly all of his baseball games and practices last season. They go fishing together, flea market hopping, play board games, practice playing baseball together.

I am so incredibly thankful for the grandfather my son has found in my father. Thankful for rest. Thankful Dom and Iz will have special memories of my father when they're older.

Monday - September 15 2014

Over the weekend, I was attempting to button one of Izzy's shirts. I struggled for a few minutes with the button. Once I actually looked at it, instead of focusing on her, I was able to get her dressed without complications.

The tingling in my fingertips has begun to spread and is worsening by the day. I can't feel the tips of them anymore where my nail is. Now the tingling sensation, followed by complete numbness, has spread to the first horizontal line on all of my fingers and both of my thumbs. It's the same with my toes. It started at the tips and has spread slowly to almost halfway down my feet. I'm so used to it now.

Explains why it was so difficult to button her shirt. I couldn't feel the button in my fingertips.

The feeling is only amplified by cold weather. I have to say, I'm pretty thrilled about chemo being done before Winter. Walking around a massive campus in forty-degree New England weather, after chemo, last semester was not fun.

Part of my chemo regimen is a drug called Oxaliplatin. One of the side effects is the tingling and numbness I've been experiencing in my hands and feet. My oncologist lowered the dose two treatments ago but this neuropathy is persistent. He's decided to cancel the Oxaliplatin dose altogether for my last treatment, scheduled for the day after tomorrow.

It may be postponed until next week. My body feels a certain way when platelets are too low for chemo. Each time I've felt chemo would be held off due to low counts, I was right. It's already happened at least a half a dozen times. I've been feeling that way again this week, but my guess is I'm borderline for treatment. I have labs in the morning, so I should know by tomorrow afternoon if I graduate from chemo this week or not.

Tuesday - September 16, 2014

Yesterday Mom and me sat out on the back patio, enjoying slightly cool weather and sunshine.

Don't remember what we spoke about. Only remember feeling happy to be spending quality time with her.

Wednesday - September 17, 2014
CHEMO SESSION # 12
FINAL TREATMENT
weight: 133.4 pounds/60.50 kilograms

What an emotional ending to an extraordinary journey. Hugs, tears and laughter were shared between me, Mom and the nurses. They never expected to see me pull out my college graduation cap for *Chemo Graduation Day* photos! Here's to the next chapter of my life. Here's to the people and adventures that await! With all ends, come new beginnings. I'm ready.

Chemo wiped me out today. Last session but not the easiest. I took advantage of Mom occupying Dom and Iz and napped for a bit. Steroids from chemo have me wired, unable to sleep more. Dad stopped by too which made it easier for Mom. I'm sure of it.

Last night I baked a huge home-made casserole dish of three-cheese, Italian, stuffed shells. Izzy helped mix the cheese, egg and other ingredients before filling the shells. Not long after that she fell asleep watching a movie. Mom left for work so once dinner was done, me and Dad sat down to eat at a table for two.

Saturday - September 20, 2014

Chemo is over. Yesterday my 48-hour chemo pump was disconnected for the last time. In the months to come, I have several follow-up appointments. There will regular check-ins with my oncologist, surgeon and gastroenterologist. In December I'll need a follow up colonoscopy to ensure the cancer hasn't come back. The next stage of my journey is just beginning. Survivorship.

Friday - September 26, 2014

Feeling energized after a Facetime chat with my "sister from another mister" and her beautiful twin babes. She's an amazing mom. Thankful for the graces of technology allowing me to witness her little ones' pure adoration toward their mama. They were listening attentively to every word she said. They would reach out here and there with a gentle hand to touch her face. Seeing the way her son looks at her, he is positively *smitten* by her!

I'm moved by her patience with them. The way she goes about feedings and playtime and diaper changes, time two, leaves me astonished. She tells me that it doesn't always work out like that, where she's able to manage everything effortlessly. What I do know with certainty is those babes are blessed to have her.

It's been nearly four years since we last spent time together in person. We've both moved, a few times, since our friendship began in Colorado seven years ago. There are hundreds of miles between us yet somehow we always find a way to be part of eachother's lives.

11
OCTOBER 2014
Purpose

"I never change,
I simply become more myself."
~Joyce Carol

Tuesday - October 21, 2014

Life is almost back to normal. My body feels stronger than it has since this cancer journey began. I've gained nearly 15 pounds since I was first diagnosed! Thankful for the weight gain. Thankful for chemo being over. Thankful for Dom sitting next to me at the table with me just now. He had his laptop, my old computer, in tow and looked at me with a mischievous smile. "Oh look at me! I'm all type-typey, nerdy-nerdy like my mom!" Then he began dramatically button mashing the keyboard keys, causing a fit of hysterical laughter between the two of us. Sitting here with Dom, watching Izzy play is the greatest gift.

Recently, I attended a book signing for *Buried Beneath the Words* by Betel Arnold. We connected instantly. There were many parallels in our lives. She saw herself in me; a young woman with hope and dreams bigger than the sky. Without blinking, she looked directly into my eyes and said, "You are destined for great things. I can see it all over you! I'm so happy for you and the path you're on. You're going to accomplish so much and I would really like to be part of it." Her words moved a mountain within my spirit. Somewhere on a deep core level, I could feel it. She was right.

12
NOVEMBER 2014
Inspiration

"Surround yourself with people who add value to your life.
Who challenge you to be greater than you were yesterday.
Who sprinkle magic into your existence, just like you do into
theirs.
Life isn't meant to be done alone.
Find your tribe, and journey freely and loyally together."
~Alex Elle

Friday - November 21, 2014
weight: 141.5 pounds/64.18 kilograms

Kim hosted a girl's night out event for me tonight! I was reminded of the many blessings in my life and the lives of my children. There were many people I knew but quite a few I met for the first time. All came out to celebrate the gift of life. She had tee shirts and tank tops made, with the words "Amber Strong" on the front and a 1950's cartoon woman flexing her muscles on the back. The thought bubble for the cartoon character read, "Fight like a girl."

This past Tuesday was Dom's first basketball practice. It was more of an introductory session. Get the kiddos together, run some drills, arrange the teams. As usual, Izzy wasn't about to sit still while all this was going on. I made an executive decision to walk with her out in the hall while Dom played in the gym.

Dom played basketball last Fall as well. I'd walk Izzy up and down the hallways of Dom's elementary school in her stroller. Up and down, forth and back we went while he practiced in the gymnasium. It was exhausting but I didn't know I had cancer yet so I thought it was normal "mom fatigue." It was tiresome maintaining the energy required to keep up with both of them.

Fast forward to basketball practice last Tuesday. Izzy was ecstatic we were going for a walk in the hall. "Mommy, let's have a race! On your mark, get set… Go!" She took off down that corridor so fast her dark brown curls bounced from shoulder to shoulder.

Izzy's raspy giggle echoed throughout the hall as I ensued. I didn't need to catch my breath. Anxiety didn't pound away at my chest with rhythmic fury. In fact, *I* was running circles around *her*! My three-year-old had to stop to catch *her* breath. We ran up the hall and back down a few more times. Izzy was exhausted but I felt ready to run a marathon! I felt alive.

I had an epiphany. My body is getting stronger every day. I feel healthier and happier as more time passes. It's been two months now since my final chemo treatment. In that moment, as all these thoughts passed through my mind, I was overwhelmed with gratitude.

My health is doing more than returning to me, it's being renewed. I feel healthier now, for the most part, than I have in over a decade. I have the energy to run circles around my children and it feels incredible!

No more sitting on the couch, for hours on end, barely able to move from sheer exhaustion. No more staying inside during the winter, unable to play in the snow with my children. The harsh cold won't cause excruciating pain against my chemo infused skin. No need to tag in my relatives for help with the kids out of necessity.

I'm not weak anymore. I'm strong. Empowered.

13
DECEMBER 2014
The Best is Yet to Come

> *"Just when the caterpillar*
> *thought the world was over,*
> *it became a butterfly…"*
> *~anonymous*

Thursday - December 11, 2014

Tomorrow is a big day. It's been nearly one year since I was diagnosed with cancer. Time for a follow up colonoscopy. Two bottles of magnesium citrate to clear everything out. No way in hell was I going to drink that gallon of chalk water again. At least having Dom here to cheer me by yelling, "Chug! Chug! Chug!" makes it far more entertaining. Re-check in the morning, fingers crossed!

Friday - December 12, 2014
Frank Sinatra's Birthday!

Just came out of my procedure. No polyps, lumps, bumps or tumors. Most importantly, no cancer! I am officially cancer free!

Yesterday morning, I began thinking about the gravity of how this colonoscopy could potentially affect my life. If it went one way, I would be deemed "cancer free" and wouldn't have to have another colonoscopy for another year. If there was something; a polyp, another tumor, a growth, unhealthy tissue; I couldn't fathom what that would have meant.

Everything went as scheduled. I arrived a few minutes late for my 7:55 a.m. check in, got changed into a hospital gown and followed the medical assistant to my hospital bed. I met with several lovely people who would be part of my procedure that morning; the anesthesiologist, the nurse who would be monitoring my vitals, another nurse who administered the IV into my port, "That is one prominent port you have there! That's wonderful!"

One of the nurses and one of the anesthesiologists whisked me away to the procedure room, gurney and all. They positioned me on my left side in the bed, as the Dr. S came into the room.

The anesthesiologist counted some deep breaths with me, slowly, in and out. Before I knew it, I woke up in the recovery room. My vision was still hazy as I came to but I overheard Dr. S speaking to my mother. There was a smile in her voice as she said, "Everything looks great! Nothing but good news to report, she did extremely well and everything is healthy and looks normal."

Mom was overjoyed. I couldn't see her yet but I heard the happiness in her voice. As she drove us home, I answered a call from Nate on my phone. "Hey Wonder Woman!" Over the last year, I could hear the concern in his voice more than once when we spoke about my treatment or diagnosis. Today though, we were talking about how well everything went. The happiness in his voice made me smile.

I'm eager to see what the future holds. I'm thankful for the present moment. My heart is full.

178

14
AFTERWORD
Grace

"Let gratitude be the pillow
upon which you kneel to say your nightly prayer."
~Maya Angelou

If you've taken time to read this book, and gotten as far as the afterword, I'd like to extend my gratitude by saying, *Thank You.* There are countless other books out there you could have chosen to read. Yet here you are, holding a piece of my life in your hands. You chose to embark on the journey of a thousand steps with me. A journey that began when I was diagnosed with Stage III Colon Cancer in 2013.

Sacred Awakening began in 2014 when I began keeping a collection of personal blog posts and journal entries of my cancer journey.

In February of 2018 it became an intense labor of love, morphing into book form, as each entry was painstakingly pieced together. It was written at all hours of the night and into the early morning. My creative muse possessed me while sitting in the grass at my daughter's soccer practice, or at a table in a book store café while Dom and Izzy were at school. Every waking moment I had, over the course of four months was spent putting this book together.

We have to make time to do the things we love. You work a nine to five? Okay, what are you doing from six to seven in the morning before you go in? You're a single mom? So am I.

It's *imperative* that we make time in our lives to let inspiration in, to align ourselves with that which ignites our souls. If we want to truly live, and not just be alive, we have to make a conscious effort to see the light even when there's darkness around us.

We all have a story. Every one of us. A traumatic event, a loved one we've lost, a personal battle of some kind. Being openly vulnerable about my cancer story has helped me help countless other people along their own journeys, long before *Sacred Awakening* was written.

When I began waking up to the world around me, I noticed the prevalence of cancer in my life. A little over a year after I finished treatment, I lost my Godmother to lung cancer. One of my cousins was diagnosed with breast cancer and one of my best friends from high school recently passed from cervical cancer.

Why are certain cancer rates so much higher in the United States than other countries of the world? I believe a huge component of that has to do with our environment. When you start to research the carcinogenic properties of chemicals found in every day household products like makeup[6], cleaners and air fresheners[7] (just to name a few) – the results are staggering.

What I realized early on in my cancer journey is that we are doing this to ourselves for the most part. Cancer, diabetes, heart disease. All of it. I understand about five to ten percent of cancer is caused by genetics. That's not what I'm referring to here.

Find a product in your home, any product that's not naturally derived. Look at the ingredient label. Pick an ingredient, probably the most difficult to pronounce, and put it into a Google search engine followed by the words "link to cancer" or "carcinogenic properties." I can almost bet you'd be shocked by the results that come up.

New scientific studies show that countless protein powders are loaded with heavy metals such as cadmium, mercury, lead and arsenic[10] – and that's across the board; organic, vegan, conventional.

Until we stop manufacturing products like aluminum based deodorant[8], makeup with parabens and polyparabens, or adding glycol and Tetra sodium EDTA[9] to our products, we are going to keep getting sick and handing money over to large corporations who make billions off of disease. We have to take charge of our health. Our wellness. Our futures.

Not everyone believes in holistic wellness. Not everyone has the opportunity to get a second opinion or can afford to eat healthier on a limited income. We all do the best with what we have and what we know at the time. The more we educate ourselves, the greater our chances of accessing a higher quality of life – a healthier way of being.

I went through major surgery. Endured eight months of chemotherapy. I battled depression, financial strain, romantic heartache and physical changes in my body. My mental state was as stable as a straw house hit by a hurricane. When I underwent treatment in 2014, it was what I have come to call "the best, worst, year of my life."

I'm here to say, well, I'm *here*. I want to speak exclusively to the newly diagnosed cancer patients, to the twenty and thirty somethings who are shocked by their recent prognosis.

You *can* do this. My hope is that you read my story and feel inspired to live your best life, on your own terms. Get a second opinion, ask tons of questions, make sure you really click with your oncologist.

I had a therapist once who told me clients don't experience positive outcomes based on the number of years a therapist has been practicing. They experience positive outcomes based on how well they connect with their therapist.

I believe the same holds true for physical ailments. It's imperative when you're going through something like cancer to have a medical team you can trust.

The doctors did their best to keep me informed throughout the course of treatment but there were several things they didn't address. Survivor's guilt, body image issues, post-traumatic stress disorder.

About 15 months after completing my last chemotherapy treatment, my Aunt Anne lost her five-year battle to Stage IV Lung Cancer. I never once asked "why me" when I was going through my own cancer battle. I did when she passed. I asked, "Why me? Why am I still here?" It triggered suppressed emotions that I hadn't given myself the space to process previously. Mainly, survivor's guilt.

In 2017, one of my dearest high school friends lost her battle to Cervical Cancer. Millie was in her early thirties. A mom of four. One of the kindest, brightest lights of a soul I have met. When she passed it made me question again, "Why me?" She *deserves* to be here. She *should* be here. Anger rose up from my belly, releasing itself through a sea of tears.

My doctors never warned me about things like that. They never told me about the self-esteem issues I would face going out in public with a tank top on. My Porta Cath prominently displayed for all to see when warm weather hit. People stared, wondering what it was.

There was a young, twenty something, sales clerk at a popular lingerie store who would always tell me how "cool looking" my implant was when I came in to shop. She was oblivious to the fact that it was for administering chemo meds.

Doctors couldn't prepare me for what cancer triggers, still, emotionally. How, years after chemo I feel uncomfortable under fluorescent lights because they trigger memories from surgeries and hospital stays. The smell of rubbing alcohol makes me nauseous from all the times I tasted it in the back of my throat before treatment.

I still haven't been able to watch the movie *The Fault in Our Stars* all the way through. My sister lent it to me one weekend toward the end of my treatment. I made it half way through before having an emotional breakdown and shutting it off. Maybe now that I'm stronger I can sit down and try to watch it all the way through. With a massive box of tissues when no one is home so I can embrace the "ugly cry" as Oprah calls it.

One of the reasons writing this book was so important to me is because unless someone has lived through it, they can't fully understand how cancer and chemo and other forms of treatment affect the mind, body and spirit.

On the outside we may look fine. On the inside we may be having suicidal thoughts, or feeling amazing or be totally confused from the brain fog of treatment. It's impossible to know for certain what someone is experiencing from the outside.

Because I didn't have a romantic partner when I was going though treatment, it caused me to seek out self-love in its purest form. When my gums were severely bleeding from low red cell counts and my hair became thinner and thinner, it was up to me to look myself in the mirror and (in my best Ryan Gosling voice) say, "Hey girl, you're beautiful. I love you. You got this." The love I had been hoping to share with Felipe or someone else, I gave to myself instead tenfold.

I did end up going on that women's retreat. It was interesting to discover that some of the things I did intuitively on my own in 2014 before the retreat; creating a playlist to shift my moods, daily exercise, gratitude, journaling – were part of the emotional tools we were given at the retreat. It did help me stick to those rituals though.

It also brought a soul sister friendship into my life, changing my entire world for the better. Cha Ching! Love you Emms! But that's a story for another book.

Looking back, there are things I would have done differently. I would have gotten a second opinion. I would have tried more holistic remedies. I would have gone to the doctor a whole hell of a lot sooner.

If you've been experiencing symptoms of any kind that feel "abnormal" no matter how small, tune in to your body and see if it feels serious. Trust your intuitive feeling. Then go to your doctor! Seriously. Guess what? Everyone goes "number two." Everyone urinates. We all have the same stuff on the inside. Not having a conversation with your doctor because *you* feel uncomfortable talking to them about bodily functions and fluids is the dumbest damn reason to not take care of yourself.

Who gives a shit what your doctor thinks about what you tell them? Honestly if they judge you and make you feel uncomfortable, it may be time to find a new doctor. Don't you deserve to have peace of mind about your own health? The answer is YES of course you do!

If you feel intuitively that something is wrong but your doctor disagrees, find another doctor or ask for more tests to be run, get a second opinion.

If you disagree with conventional remedies, seek out an alternative medicine doctor. Whatever it may look like for you, find out what's going on and then do something to help kick start the healing process.

During the three months leading up to my first colonoscopy, all kinds of tests were ordered that came back negative. A CT scan, two full panels of blood work, an ultrasound. ALL came back negative. It took finally going in for a colonoscopy to discover I had cancer the whole time.

If you're going though cancer alone, you *can* get through it. There are so many resources available if you're willing to do a little research or ask your doctors or nurses. Build your support system, however that may look for you.

Connect with your passions; reading, cooking, painting, music, nature walks or whatever you're into if none of that "nerd stuff" (as Dom refers to it) floats your boat. Remember to be kind to yourself. Give thanks for what you have and release what you have no control over.

Never stop working on yourself either. It took a few years before I was financially self-supporting after treatment ended. Cancer taught me that personal development is a life-long course we never fully graduate from. I continue to work on myself daily, over four years later. Through priming, journaling, gratitude and exercise I'm able to channel my "why" on a consistent basis.

There is unimaginable strength within us all. Through the power of gratitude, strengthened by faith and surrounded by family – I found a way to pull myself through. If *I* can do it, I know *you* can find a way too.

"Hold your head high, never let it define the light in your eyes, love yourself, give it hell, stand and be strong, never give up, conquer with love and fight like a girl."

Letter to Cancer

Dear Cancer,

You may not remember me but I will never forget you.

We met, officially, in December of 2013. You'd been watching me for some time, though only you would know how long that was before we became acquainted. Was it months? Perhaps years?

I had an inkling something wasn't right. I could feel your presence lingering around me, dropping hints, robbing my curves of their soft flesh for years, leaving behind a frame comparable to that of a pre-pubescent boy.

When you made your debut into my life that summer (2013), you didn't introduce yourself properly. You told me your name was stress. But what's in a name right? So I reserved doubt about your true nature only for conversations with overly concerned family members.

Apparently their concern was warranted.

By the time you revealed your true nature to me, you had already begun infesting my life from behind the scenes. My colon, my rectum, my lymph nodes. You were a literal pain in the ass. I thought major colon resection surgery was enough to evict your sorry ass from occupying my temple. But being the persistent little fucker you are, I was wrong.

Too many lymph nodes were tainted by your indecency and overexposure to the healthy cells in my body. So you introduced me to Chemotherapy and Steroids. I hated all of you but I never

questioned why you (Cancer) chose me. I never wondered why in all the healthy people of the world you wanted me. You're a selfish prick, why not me?

Your friend Chemo took my energy. The steroids brought insomnia, and also an unbelievably strong desire to rotate furniture and clean at 2 a.m. (Who would have guessed right?) My sleep patterns are still somewhat fucked. Being the bully you are, you taunted me by letting my hair thin just enough to make me self-conscious, but not enough for anyone else (but my hairdresser) to notice. Guess what fucker? It grew back in twice as thick and healthier than ever.

And my curves? They're back too. In one year, I've gained more weight than I could have hoped for. I fit into my jeans in all the right places. My thighs are so sexy they can't stop touching each other. I finally feel like the beautiful woman I am. The warrior. The survivor.

I should really be thanking you Cancer.

You brought me closer to my family. You've given me new found friendships that continue to change my life for the better. I'm inspiring those around me and taking better care of my mind and body than I ever thought I would. I've tapped into an inner strength that I didn't even know existed. You tried to take it all from me, but in the end Cancer, all you did was give me everything.

I know there's always that slim possibility we'll meet again someday. Just know if we do, I'll be ready for you. You've been warned.

Never or truly yours,

Amber

References

[1] *http://www.unm.edu/~lkravitz/Article%20folder/musicexercise.html*
[2] *https://www.acefitness.org/certifiednewsarticle/805/ace-sponsored-research-exploring-the-effects-of/*
[3] *https://www.healthline.com/health-news/mental-listening-to-music-lifts-or-reinforces-mood-051713#1*
[4] *https://www.healthychildren.org/English/healthy-living/emotional-wellness/Pages/Music-and-Mood.aspx*
[5] *https://www.healthychildren.org/English/healthy-living/emotional-wellness/Pages/Music-and-Mood.aspx*
[6] *https://www.beautybyearth.com/over-1000-toxic-ingredients-banned-in-europe-but-not-in-us/*
[7] *https://www.sciencedirect.com/science/article/pii/S0360132316304334*
[8] *https://www.cancer.org/cancer/cancer-causes/antiperspirants-and-breast-cancer-risk.html*
[9] *https://bubbleandbee.com/top-five-chemicals-to-avoid/*
[10] *https://www.consumerreports.org/dietary-supplements/heavy-metals-in-protein-supplements/*

I invite you to continue the conversation online
in
The Sacred Awakening exclusive Facebook
group:

https://www.facebook.com/groups/SacredAwakeningBook/